MY TWO CENTS' WORTH ON PREGNANCY

The Reality of a Future Mom

JASNA ZEKIC

Dedicated to all future moms-to-be

CONTENTS

That first pregnancy is a long sea journey to a country where you don't know the language, where land is in sight for such a long time that, after a while, it's just the horizon—and then one day birds wheel over that dark shape, and it's suddenly close, and all you can do is hope like hell that you've had the right shots.

– Emily Perkins

This memoir is about my unique nine months of pregnancy and how I dealt with the so-called "normal" side effects. With each trimester came different changes and it was not easy to get a grasp on all those challenges without complaining.

It did not make sense to complain to the men in my life or to question the most beautiful design that Mother Nature created for us. It did not make sense to complain to the women who had been through it at least once and yet somehow had forgotten all the pain as soon as the child was delivered into this world.

It made the most sense to complain to the politicians

about the social system in place to support pregnant women, but I had no strength to do that.

I could only express my discomfort by writing this book during those sleepless nights, questioning the process of child-bearing, and anticipating what the next day may bring.

To declare that I was out of my mind while under the influence of naturally producing hormones would be a reasonable statement. While walking on the borderline of insanity, any of this mumbo jumbo that I wrote while pregnant should be questionable.

In case anyone thinks this is just a lame excuse to politely cover my behind, then I challenge you to try it out for a few days or weeks and only pretend to have one or two of pregnancy's side effects.

This is a creative nonfiction tale with a lot of true lies, white lies, and plain lies, so I dare you to prove me wrong and figure out which one is which.

FIRST TRIMESTER

TAKE OFF

MONTH 1 - JUNE

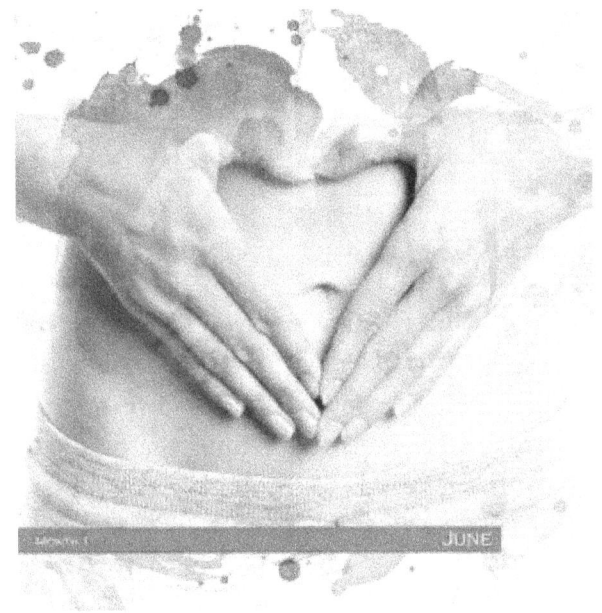

ME AS A MOM AND THE LUCKY TIMING

An interesting fact that stuck in my head for a long time from the TV programs on nature is that, on average, during an ejaculation, one man produces enough sperm to impregnate every woman in Europe. And yet, during all these years I was getting lucky, I was so lucky not to get pregnant?

Luckily it was only a good practical experience without a final product.

Why is that?

I didn't want to get pregnant. I just wanted to get lucky.

This precious thing called life is of interest to other researchers. The Goldilocks effect, the principle which describes the precise conditions that have to be met in order for life to start, is also something that has to do with a lot of luck. If not familiar with this concept, don't worry about it for now.

You are probably familiar with stories of couples' difficulties having kids, no matter how right the conditions were. No doctor could determine why the conception did not happen already. Couples are under so much stress when wanting kids, and, as soon as they forget all about it, luckily, it happens.

Is it possible and just as simple that, when a woman wants to get pregnant, she gets pregnant?

I felt lucky that I got pregnant when it happened. Most of my friends have their children almost out of the house or in their teens or at least old enough to go to school on their own.

But was I really ready to have kids in my twenties or thirties? How I felt about having a child ten years ago is a whole new chapter. I was in the comfort zone before it happened, thinking that my egg count was so low that I could have all the sex I wanted. Free sex for me, yippee.

Since I didn't get pregnant by now, then I would never get pregnant was my wrong thinking.

Bang.

I took the first home pregnancy test one month after a missed period. A positive test would show two lines in a small area, with a negative being only one line. The results of the first test were one clearly visible line and one half-ass visible line just barely showing.

I decided to redo the test the next morning, check if that line gets thicker or weaker on the old test, and compare it to the new test. Maybe it was also my mind playing tricks on me, and I wanted to see what I wanted to see.

For about two decades, I was more in a preventive mode when it came to pregnancy than in a proactive mode of visiting doctors and trying to get pregnant. That story is to be told at some other time, but I just wanted to touch on it, so it is clear why my mind may have had a reason to play tricks on me, for me to believe that I was not pregnant. We all know that life changes, but, at the same time, I had no good reason for being scared to death and totally flipping out if it were true that I was pregnant.

My life is much more stable and secure now than it was twenty years ago, so it can't be that horrible to get pregnant right now. Plus I have always said, if and when I do get pregnant, then of course my choice would be to have the child. An abortion was out of the question.

The next day the test showed two equally thick lines.

BOY, BOY, BOY, BOY. SURE I AM SURE.

I am sure there are better ways of waking up my boyfriend with this big news than the way I did.

"How about an omelet for breakfast with coffee? By the way I am pregnant."

It didn't happen exactly like that, but I delivered the news without any creativity and during his first waking minutes.

"It's a boy," he said. He had had a dream before I woke him up and was convinced our baby was a boy.

The most interesting fact that happened in coming weeks and months was that, all of a sudden, anywhere I went, I saw pregnant women, as if they hadn't existed before. They were everywhere, I tell ya. If the woman was not pregnant, she had a baby in a stroller.

I could have bet you money that, every time, the baby was a boy. I could make my bets high, because I would win the money. The baby was always a baby boy. At the doctor's office or at the grocery store, shopping mall, or on a bus, boys were running everywhere.

I even came up with my own conspiracy theories. How can that be? So many kids and yet so many boys? Is there something in the water that we should know about? Maybe the government is doing some kind of an experiment on us? Is WWIII coming, and we need many more men to fight it? Of course these were all my silly jokes. None of them could qualify as a conspiracy theory, but, not even up to the date of this writing, can I explain the probabilities of baby boy occurrences in the first three months of my pregnancy.

I also wanted a boy. Why?

If I describe myself in terms of how girlie girl I am, on a scale from zero to ten, with number ten being as girlie girl as one can get, then I would say my number is one. Barely enough to qualify as a girl.

If I have a daughter and that means we have to match our outfits and do her hair and buy pink skirts and play with dolls—well, yeah, then I am in trouble. Or, worse yet, my little girl is in trouble, because most of my answers would sound like this:

"Yeah, that looks good. Let's go now. We are late."

Or …

"What do you need that dress for? You already have one like that at home."

My little girl would lose out, if she had it in her nature to dress neatly, to match everything, because her mama does not have a taste or a desire for what it takes to be a girlie girl.

With a boy, on the other hand, I know what to do. Buy a couple casual outfits, a dozen T-shirts and jeans, a bunch of sneakers and balls, and tell him to go play soccer with his father.

I told my boyfriend about this plan of mine, the grand master plan that I have, so we can just even out the responsibilities here. For all the hard work I am doing now and the suffering I am going through for the next nine months, it is only fair to give the child to the father, as soon as he is born, telling Dad, "Honey, I did my part. Now you deal with him."

I did not want to hear any of this *Mama, Mama, Mama* business.

Daddy should be his word of choice. The first word too and, after that, it will be *Daddy, Daddy, Daddy*.

ON YOUR MARK! READY, SET, AND GROW!

Have you ever wondered what the world would look like if every pregnant woman stopped working during her entire pregnancy?

We all have our different ways of doing things, and pregnancy can be a complicated matter to reveal. Many women wait for three months to declare their pregnancy to the world. Some don't say anything until others notice her swelling stomach and start asking questions. For me it was not so easy to find the right timing, and I ended up just blurting it out while at work ...

"This concludes our meeting, and, ah, ... oh, ... by the way, I am pregnant."

I could hardly pronounce those words.

Kitty got your tongue? You could say that. I just could barely do it.

I kept it a secret as long as I could.

THE MOTHER OF ALL ULTIMATE CHALLENGES

I have a challenge! If you have never been pregnant, you should try it out sometime or at least pretend to be. Whether a man or a woman, it doesn't matter. Just like kids get a school assignment to take care of a chicken egg for a week and pretend it was a baby, we can simulate the side effects for this pregnancy task and pretend.

Would you like to accept the challenge for a day, a week, or a month? Without knowing the side effects?

Here is the first challenge. You choose a trimester—select first, second, or third.

For the first trimester, we will give you the following side effects:

On a particular day you get a bloated stomach, constipation, the headache, and loss of appetite. We may surprise you and make it last for a few hours or days. Also a nasty combination of all side effects could last for a few weeks.

Here are the quick instructions for dealing with your bloated stomach.

Hold it all in.

Don´t just think you can get rid of that stinky gas any time you wish or at any place.

No, sir.

I also wondered how my body could produce such a stink and the same goes for the smell of my urine. My gosh! I swear, up to this day, I still cannot figure out what the contents, what the ingredients could possibly be to smell like that.

How would you like to sleep for months with growing pressure on your bladder? A pressure that you don´t know if it's an infection of your bladder, uterus, or ovaries, or some odd combination of all three. Who cares, right? Just please, pain, go away.

Here is an additional challenge for you, since it looks like you are able to handle this pretty well. How about I challenge you to have eight hours of complete energy depletion, and you have only enough energy to go to bed?

Sorry, what bed? You are at the workplace and, of course, expected to produce deliverable outcomes. *Bed* in your dreams maybe but not now, so sleep on someone else´s time.

Oh, you are losing your voice because you are so tired?

Well, too bad. Just whisper.

We will bring you a microphone too, if we can´t hear you.

In case you have forgotten what a workplace can be, let me redefine it for you. It is a place of written rules of expectations on unwritten behaviors. A world of hidden ethical rules with unwritten laws that can only get you if you disobey them. The person with a higher authority than yours has every right to apply any of those unwritten rules against you. That´s a definition of a workplace for you.

What are you going to tell them?

"Give me a break. I am pregnant."

Oh, yeah, the wolves would love to hear that excuse, so they could eat you and the baby alive.

Or better yet, you lose your cool and end up with a short fuse and say something as dumb as:

"I quit."

Not now, buddy. You can´t quit now, when you need those health benefits to cover the hospital bills and the half-ass compensation after the baby is born. You bet your sweet ass that you will suck it up to any kind of a boss you may have and do it with a smile.

I better quickly add the (unnecessary) disclaimer that I have the best boss in the whole world.

COFFEE WITHDRAWAL–OR IS IT?

Coffee addiction is nothing new to me! Let´s not underestimate "guzzling" as a word choice when it came to my daily consumption.

"Next in line please!"

"Hi."

"Good morning."

"What can I get for you, ma'am?"

"One gallon of coffee to go please!"

Before the pregnancy, at times, it counted as breakfast, and other times it counted as dinner. Skipping a meal was not a big deal because of this tasty beverage that can trick the appetite.

Going cold turkey with coffee causes withdrawals. One of the known side effects is headaches. This was my case too, and I could not tell the difference between the headaches from my pregnancy with its hormone changes and the coffee withdrawals. A headache is a headache. It didn't matter.

During the first few dry days, that was not the only dirty side effect. I had bigger issues. It was the urge to argue. I started to snap, talk back, and I didn't know when to stop. Can I really blame coffee withdrawal for having the urge to argue for about a month? I doubt it.

Luckily, during one of my doctor's visits, I was informed that having two cups of coffee per day with milk is allowed during my pregnancy.

"You keep the milk, Doc. I'll have it straight!"

That first cup! Oh, joy; oh, joy. It was so wild, as if I was a bit high.

Did my desire to argue stop?

What do you think?

The best doctors in the world would have a hard time determining if my filthy mood to argue was caused only by one source or a cocktail of many factors. Hormone changes with the combination of sleepless nights, dehydration, and exhaustion can make any nice person turn into a barbaric and intolerable character.

That's my story, and I'm sticking to it!

WHAT KIND OF A BITCH AM I TODAY?

Not to give a bad name to any of the dog types, but, if I were to compare my mood to the mood of a dog, I wonder which breed I would end up being? I hate to use this comparison, since each dog has a different character, just the way women do. But, just for fun, I took an online test to compare a match with my pregnancy mood of the day to a dog type.

So the test goes like this (borrowed from dog-types.com), with my input information as follows:

- Energy level – low.
- Exercise requirements – high.
- Playfulness – medium.
- Affection level – low.
- Friendly toward other people – low.
- Ease of training – low.
- Watchdog ability – high.
- Protection – high.
- Grooming required – low.
- Cold and hot tolerance – medium.

The results gave a half-dozen breeds and types, some of which I'd never heard of before. My choice was a Dandie Dinmont terrier. The terrier part is more like a bad typo for *terror*, or, simply to break it down and translate for you, it means to tear you apart.

That´s my bitchy mood for today.

Do you feel lucky to ask any questions inside my current dog territory?

Woof!

SMOKING ROOMS, PRAYER ROOMS, AND RESTROOMS

In the first month of my pregnancy, I was so supertired that, on one occasion, I ended up in the company's medical department. So there I was, jolly me, expecting to get some kind of special treatment, if I just make a simple announcement:

"I am pregnant and feeling a little tired right now."

The way the lady looked at me from behind the front desk made me realize that I was not due any special treatment.

"So, how can I help you?"

I asked if they had a rest area in their department, where I could just lie down for twenty minutes. The answer was no, unless this was an illness related to the job. I asked if there was a wellness program in the company and if they offered a yoga class or anything of that sort.

"Yes, there is a yoga class offered for company personnel,

but it is held outside the company premises, and it starts after 6:00 p.m. on certain days."

What I heard is every second Tuesday during the month of February in a leap year.

"There is no yoga mattress anywhere on site, so I could just meditate for ten minutes and get my energy going?"

Negative again. *Wonderful*, I was thinking, while leaving this phony woman. Wait a minute. Should I go back and say what's on my mind?

No, no, no. Something is wrong here when each large building in this company has a smoking room and not one square yard as a rest area. I am aware of at least ten smoking rooms for every building I had visited for business purposes. The owners have even opened up a new one, specially built from ground zero, just outside the company's cafeteria. So if you want to smoke, we can help you support that nasty habit and accommodate you with a specially designated area.

If you want to just sit and relax without a cigarette in your hand, then you have to go home and claim that you are not feeling well due to a personal illness.

I hadn't even asked the breast-feeding questions yet, but I think I'll pass on those. It's better that I do not even try to have that discussion with this artificial person.

A few days later I made my way to the company's insurance carrier, just down the road from my office building.

"Hi, I am pregnant and would like to find out if there is a rest area anywhere."

"No, madam."

In this same building there was also a family and occupational services office, which offered the administrative answers but no rest area.

I told the lady that her office looked comfortable enough for me to rest a bit.

"I could lie down in that corner, because it has a nice carpet. May I?"

She agreed that it could have been utilized as such, but unfortunately she worked only until 11:00 a.m. After lunch, her office was just simply locked.

What a waste of space and my time.

My next move was to seek the religious sects to see if I could join one. It didn't matter which one at this point. Maybe in this huge international company where I worked, someone had the urge to pray or meditate, so maybe there was a prayer room. Unfortunately anyone working in a nice business suit was well paid in this company and on top of their career, so they must not have a need to pray.

The last option I had was to remodel the ladies' restroom and somehow hide in the three-square-yard space without anyone noticing me. I was not successful in carrying out this idea nor did I have a desire to be present in the commonly shared space where women do their business.

So how did I survive those days? I just had to suck it up. As everyone knows, walking is an easy exercise that gives a person energy, so that's what I ended up doing—walking away my tiredness and pretending that I was busy doing something business-related, like carrying a piece of paper as if I were delivering something to somebody.

I'LL TAKE A RAIN CHECK ON THAT

Smoking kills!

Surgeon general, blah, blah, blah!

Smoking during pregnancy causes defects in the child, blah, blah, blah.

Alcohol, blah, blah, blah.

Do warning signs really warn anyone of anything if the person does not want to be warned, even in this case while pregnant?

Can anyone stop a pregnant woman from smoking and drinking if the woman just simply doesn't care?

Have you ever seen a woman huffing and puffing on that cigarette, smoking away her own unborn child's health? You can't do a damn thing about it. If it is a friend or a stranger, it doesn't matter. The woman can do her thing and hide it too. She knows damn well what she is doing.

Or does she?

What happens as a result of her self-satisfaction, if it can even be called that in this case?

Let´s skip the child´s development inside her womb and the lack-of-oxygen part and also the underweight effects on the baby. Let´s not get into the birth defects either and, instead, get all scientific about it.

We are jumping now into the first months after the birth and doing a fast forward into the first few years of the child´s growth. The smoking women could breast-feed but the mother's milk would contained tar and other toxic substances that just don't fit into a newborn baby's nutrition requirements. How many days of work will that woman have to miss so she can take her child to the emergency room or to simply stay at home because the kid develops a flu every time someone sneezes on him/her, hence the lack of a good immune system?

Statistics tell us that the children from smoking moms usually have respiratory problems and, in many cases, asthma. Will any of these women sit down their children when they start school or during the teen years and admit:

"Sorry, baby, that you are not the number one and will never be number one in your favorite sport because you have asthma.

"Sorry, baby, that you will have to use inhalers during halftime to catch your breath.

"Sorry, baby, that your mama's bad smoking habit is the cause of your low performance."

Will that same mama tell the child about secondhand smoke after the birth, because she refused to stop smoking inside the house or the car?

Will that mama ever tell her little one how many doctor's visits were related to coughing, difficulty breathing, and problems sleeping at night, all brought on by her smoking habit?

Will her insurance rate increase every year, because her doctor bills are getting higher and higher—like they do on your car, if you were a more reckless driver every year?

I don't want to be a mama like that.

I want to breast-feed.

The kid never has to be a number one jock and the sportiest in the school, but he/she will have a chance. All those days that I will not use and abuse while the child is growing up should be credited to me right now, paid in advance.

I would like a rain check on that now please.

Why do I need it?

Because I am tired.

If you still don't understand, then let me tell you a little more on what I think about women working while pregnant.

POTTY BUSINESS AND SLEEPLESS NIGHTS

What do you know about those sleepless nights in the first trimester as a result of frequent trips to the toilet?

No matter how many boring books a pregnant woman can have on her nightstand that can help her go back to sleep, there are still those nights when she just simply cannot sleep after that third or fourth trip to the bathroom.

Yes, you read that right. Four trips in an eight-hour period of supposed sleep means a pregnant woman is getting up to go to the bathroom every two hours at night.

She is falling back to sleep only minutes before the alarm goes off, and it's time to get her sleepy head out of bed and get ready for work. To be so tired due to lack of sleep, somewhat cranky, and looking rough, while creating another human being, is not so easy while keeping the pregnancy a secret for now.

Mother Nature sure knows how to prepare a future mom for a newborn with this trick of ridiculously frequent trips to the toilet. That is the only reasonable explanation I could come up with for why pregnant women have to endure so many toilet trips in the middle of the night.

Is the baby's biorhythm already training Mama for 2:07

a.m. breast-feeding sessions? Why else would I be up at that time? Get used to being wide awake at that time, so, after the baby is born and cries at that exact time, the mom is already programmed to get up automatically.

A few months later I was fully trained and wide awake at that exact time. It was a big challenge to decide what to do during those hours before getting up for work. The list of creative things to do was interesting during the first few weeks, but, after a month of exhaustion, I didn't even care anymore to be productive and to use those hours wisely. Just staring in the dark was a good time-killer.

Here are some of my own activities done in the middle of the night: read, meditate, bake, eat, cook dinner for the following day, toss around on the couch or in the bed, watch morning-hour TV shows, check what's new on the Internet news, email someone in a different time zone and wait for an answer.

And, believe me, no matter how interesting the time-killing activity may be one night, it will get really boring after a few nights. I was different now and not the same normal person after so many sleepless nights. I am surprised that I didn't start hallucinating, since that's a possible side effect from the lack of sleep.

How would you like me as your coworker?

CONTROL YOUR WATER FLOW

If you think you have read enough about my potty business, I don´t blame you, and you are welcome to skip this section. Unless you are a nerd and like the laws of physics, then, in that case, you are not only required to read this section but you must also send me the answer to this unsolved mystery after you complete the puzzle.

So let's first review quickly what we know and start with the simple facts …

According to a mass balance theory, if the flow into the tank is equal to the flow out of the tank, then the tank is said to be in a mass balance. The conservation law of mass states that mass cannot be generated or destroyed.

My body has proven that, if I go to the bathroom and empty my "tank," the water can be regenerated within two minutes. Therefore I have proven that some parts of my body are a reactor and not a tank. I also get a feeling that I can go again and again, and empty more than during the previous trip.

Did I say that I can go again and drain my "tank" as soon as the tank was empty? And this is not a one- or a two-drop thing I am talking about. We are talking gushes and flows.

Are you still with me?

Let´s continue.

The first step in engineering is to understand the problem. So, if I got this mass balance theory correct, that would mean decreasing the flow into the tank should then decrease the flow out of the tank.

Maybe it's right in theory, but it's wrong in actual practice. Think again, engineers. If I were a theoretical physicist, then maybe these bathroom visits would be more interesting, seen as violating the laws of physics.

My rule was to stop drinking water by 10:00 p.m. and to empty my bladder before bedtime at least three times. So no food or liquid would enter the plane of my body for at least eight hours before it would be time to get up in the morning.

You can calculate how many times I went to the bathroom during the night. C'mon now, if you were paying a little attention, then you would not be giving a wild guess. The answer is four, because I already told you that I was getting up every two hours.

If I sound as if I have a bit of a cocky attitude, then my apologies. I was hoping we could move on to the real problem of where all the water comes from.

Because, if you do have the answer, then you should publish it. This could help out pregnant women everywhere by keeping them out of the bathrooms at night so they could get more rest. And think of all the embarrassing moments you could save women at work, when the only time in a week they see the boss—or should I say, when he sees them—is entering or exiting the bathroom.

Maybe you can get rich by helping others have a better understanding of this water production phenomenon. In a poor country perhaps, a plant could be genetically modified to make water and hydrate crop fields.

Thank you, hormones, for boosting my fantasy world.

I definitely need help.

WE ARE TIRED, SO GIVE US A BREAK

My female doctor instructed me to give her some kind of a sign before I was so burned out that I may even end up in the hospital with exhaustion. I didn't wait too long to give her that sign. As a matter of fact, it was easy. I broke down crying.

She got the biggest hug, after she gave me seven days of sick leave, because resting at home instead of the hospital was a preference.

From my experience in the USA, you pretty much have to be dying before a doctor voluntarily prescribes sick days. I don't know if they are afraid of the insurance companies or the employers or what. But, for sure, they are not afraid to send their sick patients back to work with the flu. Who cares that your coworkers will also get sick because of you?

Just imagine how I felt now, to have a doctor who is doing the total opposite.

If you wonder why so many pregnant women walk around at work with a big stomach and wait until the last day of their pregnancy to take leave, it's because of the system and the limited number of sick days. Well, it's because they want to be paid on leave too, so if you abuse the sick days, then the pay is decreased to that magic number of 67 percent of the salary. This is how it currently works in Germany.

Shame on the system.

Where is a lawyer when you need one, to represent the coming little one?

He/she is tired too, because it takes a lot of energy to grow, but Mama is busy and wouldn't stay still. Does anyone care? Why is it that people make a big deal about the way pregnant women behave? They are too ready to criticize these women.

When the system is the cause of it, then why does everyone keep quiet?

No, people, it is not supposed to work like that. Listen up, cats! And hear me good! We pregnant women are tired, so stop pretending to ignore the issue. Watching your own body bloat up to the point that you cannot even put on your shoes without getting tired or having pains is a real fact.

Or losing your breath while talking, because that takes too much energy out of you, is also a real fact. Losing your voice by the end of a workday is also a fact, because every ounce of your energy is sucked up in the development of a human.

To grow organs is a skill automatically programmed in our genes. I know that. It is not that I am doing something consciously and trying to take credit for it. However, to fuel those genes for the first time with inexperience is laborious.

Do you know what's the other fucky part?

The time away from work after the baby is born, if the woman decides to take unpaid leave, is counted against the number of years in service. That time away gets subtracted, and that's how much more you have to work toward your retirement. So if you are still appreciating the good ole system, think again.

Go, system, go! (Go to Hell!)

PREGNANCY UNITED

I know my bitching and whining was probably loud enough, but that will not change anything if I don't continue provoking you, so maybe you feel sorry for and have more sympathy toward pregnant women and decide to do something about it. So I have to raise some questions:

- Where are all the pregnant women and how come they have not been fighting for more maternity rights?
- Where the heck are the lawyers when you need one, to protect the tired unborn babies?

Moms forget the pain of labor and everything that they have been through as soon as the baby arrives. It is the beginning of times of joy with the baby. The little one gives a different kind of pleasure, so moms don't have time to think any more about pregnant women's rights.

Ok, fine, the women are tired and can't think straight. I can accept that.

I am still going back to my earlier question: if every woman stayed at home during her pregnancy, what would happen? When the pilots go on strike with the other transportation workers, they usually end up with the benefits they have been striking for.

Pregnant women should also go on strike, month after month. Fine, the impact on the insurance companies—or any company that now loses the manpower for so many months—would be humongous. But they could plan and budget for that.

I think the lawmakers are beating around the bush too much. Honestly I don't think anyone gives a shit about moms-to-be, and yet, somehow, these women figure out how to make the ends meet on that 67 percent pay after childbirth.

How much would my company suffer if someone was to replace me while I was spending a few extra months with my baby?

Would the police lock us up too if we got out of hand while protesting and asking for better work conditions while pregnant?

What's wrong with just letting the women work at least part time?

Can we let a pregnant woman work when she feels like it and has the energy for it?

Do you think I like showing up at the office and acting like a bitch and spreading my mood germs on others? No, not really. Even that takes up too much energy.

There should be an out-of-office reply for my emails and also a printed message from me to be handed out at the office's front doors that would say:

"Having quiet time, please leave me alone!"

Or …

"I am tired, and I don't know what to do with myself."

Or …

"Enter at your own risk."

I would definitely give a new dictionary definition on pregnancy: *frequent trips to the doctor's office, frequent trips to the bathroom, saying good-bye to a good night's sleep, visiting shopping malls because my clothes don't fit anymore, fearful about the baby's development, fearful of delivery, fearful of the world I am bringing my baby into, fearful of genes in the family "pool," and other things that I may end up dealing with that are out of my control.*

Yeah. Try to deal with all that in your head while staying calm at your desk, looking professional.

That´s why it´s time for a change.

THE RULES ON MATERNITY LEAVE ARE NOT YOUR FRIEND

When it is the time for maternity leave, let´s do the calculation of how much money one would get during the paid time away from work.

Maternity leave in Germany is treated as workers comp and short-term disability, so there is that magic number of 67 percent of the salary that one receives during the time away from work. Hey, that sounds good. I can get used to that money while not working and spending time with my baby. If there was a way to stretch that for a few years, I could really have a nice relaxing time with my child while the kid grows up.

Wrong.

There is a limit on the time and the money.

If you have a low-paying job, you get your 67 percent of that sorry-ass paycheck. But if you are in a low-to-middle-class-income bracket with a good-paying job and a decent salary, then that 67 percent does not apply to you, because it is above the maximum limit.

So you are stuck with a sum that someone calculated is good enough. Let me guess. It was probably a man who decided how much is enough for a woman and her kid.

It's not child alimony, so take it easy, buddy. Let me get my 67 percent.

It looks like no one cares that you are a successful woman with twenty years working your career and two university degrees. The salary that you are getting is not something that just happened overnight. It took years and years to get to that point, which is still just the low-to-middle-income-class or just a middle-class salary. But it doesn't matter. That's not the point.

The point is that the system wins in the end, and now you have to get used to less than that 67 percent of your paycheck. It could be less than half of your current take-home pay or whatever that max limit is. It's so wrong.

Of course more than half of that will go for the bills, rent, and other monthly payments that are now becoming a headache to you, which was never an issue before.

MONTH 2 - JULY

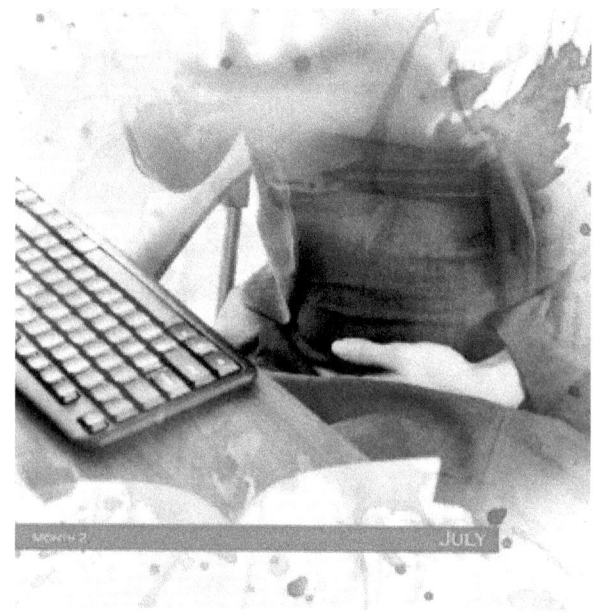

SEX DURING PREGNANCY?
NOT SO FORBIDDEN FRUIT.

The fact is that sex does not hurt the baby. Here is my theory on why Mother Nature made things so beautiful that couples can continue having sex during the pregnancy. That is, if the couple is lucky enough that the woman's hormones are stable and didn't turn her into a spider woman ready to bite the head off her man at the mention of sex.

So how come it is doable? Do you have a wild guess?

My two cents on this one is based on the evolution and the survival of the fittest:

To keep Baby's daddy around long enough. Papa is there not so much to help baby mama lift heavy things during the pregnancy. His role is to be there and help with the child's development after the birth. If he had to roam around the village and look for a piece of ass somewhere else, then he would probably never come back, and baby mama would be on her own with the baby's development. There would be less of us around.

Not that it matters to Mother Nature what kind of animal she keeps around to stay in balance.

FIRST TRIMESTER – HAIRY BUSINESS, I TELL YA

Most of my difficulties in dealing with pregnancy's side effects happened in the first trimester. I should save me some typing and gave it an abbreviation.

What do you think?

Should I call it first-T (first tee)?

Or first tree? Since it felt as if it took the same amount energy as it does growing a tree.

Is *trimester* same as *try me stir*?

Second trimester can be called *try 2 master*.

All three trimesters together: one through three. One, two, three, test, test.

So let me tell you about one interesting observation during my first-T, and this one has to do with hair depletion. Of course it was a positive phenomenon when you consider that less frequent leg-shaving was required.

If this was a story of my lawn and not my hair (wink, wink), then I would show the pictures of before and after. It is not like grass is wanted in the first place. That's why we keep on trimming and cutting. I would not pretend that I miss the weeds nor am I complaining about not having to use a weed whacker. I am only comparing a jungle with the small patches of grass, that's all. A beautiful tropical rain forest for the lack of words to convey a drought in a California golf course.

Wait a minute. I know what the presence of estrogen does during a normal monthly cycle for women, and I am aware of days of boldness. Thanks to my engineering background, and thinking in terms of mass and energy conservation, I came to a realization.

The hair must be going somewhere.

The baby. Oh, the baby is growing hair.

In my case, the baby is a child of mixed genes from two different races. Bingo. The baby is growing a fro. No wonder I wouldn't need a haircut for the next six to eight weeks.

I was wrong of course. Babies do not grow hair that early during the pregnancy, but it was the protein out of my body that was needed somewhere. Protein to grow more important things than hair, such as organs.

HELL? I CAN GIVE YOU HELL. FOR NOTHING. ABSOLUTELY FREE OF CHARGE.

The first trimester. What a beast. It needs to be locked up. It's a lethal weapon, and no woman should walk around concealing this weapon. There should be a law requiring women to have a visible sign showing they are in the first trimester. No, not on their forehead. Why is that not such a good idea? Because of the close proximity needed by the reader of the sign. By the time one realizes the bitch is pregnant, it may be too late, and the guy is history.

Pregnant women should be wearing a warning, a flashing sign with fluorescent lights, spinning and changing colors, so it cannot be confused and mistaken for any other hazardous signs. Maybe even paint the woman's face in a different color, like green or purple.

I read some time ago that, in the States, white people used to intentionally cross on the other side of the street to avoid passing a black person on the same part of the sidewalk.

My two cents on it? The pregnant woman should be painted with some glow-in-the-dark color. In case another person does not have the guts to approach this woman, the color warning should give them enough time to change to the opposite sidewalk, or to even turn around and pretend as if they have forgotten something, so they need to go back.

You know the routine. Do the whole act with the hand motions or pounding on the head when people forget something. Anything to save their ass from facing a pregnant woman.

Why am I mentioning this?

I feel that, with a little bit of legislation, the world could be a better, safer place.

I am only trying to protect the innocent, especially the men, who have no choice but to be around their pregnant *wifeee*. If someone sees a couple fighting on the streets, they could come rescue the poor guy from the lioness, if they knew she is in her first-T.

I have a story and a confession to make …

My boyfriend is a mellow guy, easygoing, and can control his rage. The total opposite of me.

It was a warm sunny day, and the evening was perfect for a walk in nature. We took a little getaway trip, just for this reason, to have the woods, the river, a quiet place to relax, and a walk in a new environment. If I described how perfect everything was, I could probably win a Nobel Prize in Literature, as long as I didn't mention my little incident in this lovely place.

I snapped. I yelled. I dramatized everything over nothing. And it wasn't only one issue that bothered me which I tripped about. I started mentioning small things that may have happened a few days or weeks or even a few months ago.

My man was speechless.

I was out of breath. That's how hard I wanted to yell but didn't have the energy to do it. The hormones were busy changing my body to make another body, but my emotions were busy changing someone else's opinion.

So what do you think is harder to do?

Well, of course it is harder to change someone's opinion to prove my own point while I am dead wrong and pregnant. I ended up with abdominal pain. Tears in my eyes.

My best friend, my boyfriend, was not so happy being next to me.

CAN THE UNBORN CHANGE A WOMAN?

It was only wishful thinking that I'd become a nicer person during my pregnancy. I snap easily if something or someone gets on my nerves, even if it's an old woman who just pushed me a little aside in a grocery store.

Plus I would make fun of everything and everybody. I would also make fun of the people or their situations just for the sake of a good joke. If a country was too small, I could make a joke out of it, or, if a guy's T-shirt was too large, I could make fun out of that too.

It wasn't even funny sometimes to some people, especially if the joke was about another culture or a political joke, and a person on the other side was sharing a different opinion. At times many people took me the wrong way, and that's only because they didn't have a sense of humor to realize it was only a joke.

So why would I put myself at risk of a verbal attack, accused and labeled? Because, to me, it was spontaneous. It was not because, down at the bottom of my heart, there was a mean person. The real reason I was doing it was only for the fun of it and to share some laughs together, if you did not take anything personal.

So that was my nature before, and it was the same during

my pregnancy. Why did I think that I could just change in a matter of days or months, just because I am pregnant?

It didn´t happen.

Yes, it would be nice not to have so many things get on my nerves. It would be ever nicer not to react to them so quickly. By the time I figured out that I had offended someone, it was too late, and the damage was already done.

If I had ten big paper clips on Friday afternoon before leaving the office, and, on Monday morning, I had nine big ones and one small one, then how many seconds does it take before my blood pressure is too high and I feel like accusing someone for taking one big paper clip and substituting it for a small one?

Ha!

How many did you guess?

Two seconds?

Luckily only two hours of negative thinking passed before the tenth paper clip was discovered under the desk, and I realized that there was no reason for this blown-out-of-proportion, unnecessary thinking.

WRITE A NOVEL. NO THANKS. I QUIT.

Where did I get the courage to start writing a book at night while having a full-time day job?

Now let me see how to go about answering this provoking question. *Beep!* Time is up. No answer. Next question. Am I on drugs? Should I go ahead and drug-test myself just to check and make sure I am not really high on something, without even knowing it? Maybe there is something in the water or in the air?

What gave me this crazy idea to write a book has nothing to do with drugs. There was more than one reason. I needed to shift my thinking to *how am I going to fall back asleep and be ready for work the next day?* I was tired of reading about pregnancy in the middle of the night; I wanted to write about it.

It was the only way to stop my bitching and whining by accepting that everything I am experiencing during my pregnancy was normal. It was time to make fun of it.

What's the worst thing that can happen if I start writing?

Oh, gee. As usual, when people are scared of something while taking up a new challenge, there is usually no need for it. So nothing bad can happen if I start writing. Absolutely nothing. It doesn't matter how far I get and if this ends up a failed project. It doesn't matter if this is a short thing with a little bit of scribbling on paper, or pages and pages of writing. Still, there should not be any bad consequences. Even if it ends up in the trash. Whoop-de-do.

So, for the fun of it, I made a table comparing writing to having a child. This Top Ten list is supposed to increase my self-esteem and encourage my ego not to give up. There should not be one good reason as a showstopper that would prevent me from writing.

Only when I think about it, am I scared. That fear disappears quickly, because I don't want to think about it. I don't think I am good at controlling my thoughts and can just say to myself, *Oh, don't think about it,* and then I would stop worrying.

Am I scared of having a child? Heck yeah.

What really makes the anxiety disappear is my love for this child and my anticipation to see and hold the baby.

Same with writing. My love for writing makes me stop thinking about what I will write about it. I just don't want to forget my experience of having this baby as soon as he is welcomed to our world. So, when in doubt, write and keep on writing.

Just love it, and that's all there is to it. Just love it.

Writing	Having a Child
1. Never wrote a book before.	1. Never gave birth before.
2. Don´t even know what to call the book.	2. Don´t even know what to call the book.
3. Never read a book on how to write a book.	3. No book can prepare me for having a child; better get my feet wet.
4. True authors get inspired by anything and get the ideas how to create something out of nothing.	4. Unbelievable moms also create something and everything from nothing for their children.
5. I speak three languages, and, no matter which one I write in, I always sound like a foreigner.	5. All foreigners know how to speak the language of love to their children. Any fool can translate the love (in writing), including a computer program.
6. To make a No. 1 seller nowadays, most books are written as fiction, and I don't even read those novels.	6. Your child will always be No. 1 to you, regardless how others label him/her (mysterious, creative, or romantic).
7. I may get a good start and soon after run out of ideas and slow down, or just do a really crappy job.	7. Do parents ever stop being parents or run out of ideas on how to stop a child from crying or how to give sloppy love? (Side joke, if you do a crappy job with this one, just have another child.)
8. If I was taking a writing class and had one month of homework to do late every night, as usual, I would do each and every one of the assignments without ever thinking ahead about what it would take to complete them.	8. Everything a child needs, every wish, will be fulfilled no matter how difficult it is or what time of the day it is.
9. What if I run out of stuff, there is no flow, and it is just simply a boring piece of work?	9. What if I run out of stuff, there is no flow, and it is just simply a boring piece of work?
10. Others will write better than me and have their No.1 sellers, but the feeling of completing a book no one can take away from me.	10. Others will write better than me and have their No.1 sellers, but the feeling of completing a book no one can take away from me.

MONTH 3 - AUGUST

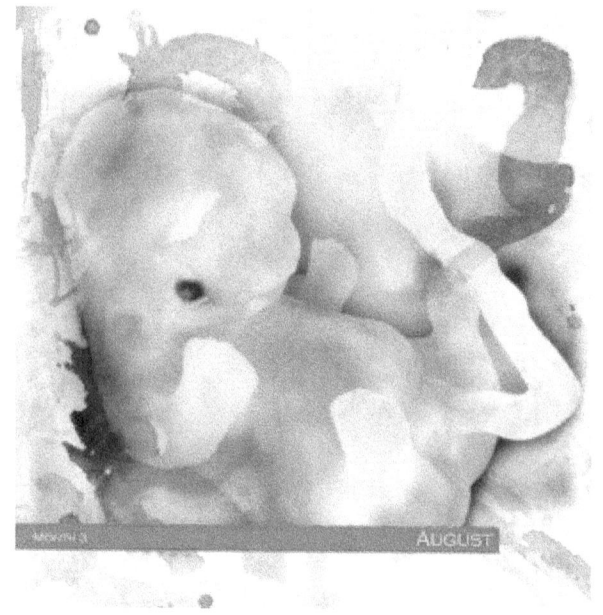

DON'T COUNT ALL YOUR CHICKENS BEFORE THEY HATCH

One reason I kept my pregnancy a secret at first was for the same reason most couples do.

Miscariage.

Scary thing! Especially at my age, with the associated risks. Most of my close friends live elsewhere, so it was easy to keep the secret. There was a good chance that none of my friends would see me in my first trimester, because they are almost on the other side of the planet, and trips to this side of the world are not so frequent.

I was not in the mood to answer anyone's questions in the first trimester. I was still busy absorbing this life-changing event and dealing with the side effects. Posting my status every day on Facebook during the early stages of my pregnancy was not my style.

Why? Because.

Because, what if something happens to the baby's development? What if there was an early complication?

What if … ?

Of course people would feel sorry for me and the baby. They would ask questions, call, and write emails to help comfort me. That's what friends are there for. I still kept quiet.

My boyfriend was supportive in this decision, but, once my belly bump started to show, we decided to tell.

What a joy that was.

LET THE PREGNANT WOMAN EAT

In the first few months, if you are lucky enough to hold down food, there may be also periods of lack of appetite and periods of lack of energy to consume anything. The only amount of energy left in a pregnant woman's body is to lie down at the end of the workday.

The hunger may still be there, but it would take too much out of her body to prepare anything or to go around the corner and get a quick bite. Therefore, don't begrudge a pregnant woman a "huge" lunch, when you don't realize she's too tired to eat dinner later that same day.

My two cents on it is that the calorie count should have a different formula between the trimesters. In the first trimester, the calories should not even count. Let the woman eat whatever she wants to eat, especially at the end of the first trimester. If the total calorie count in one day is two times greater than the daily recommended amount, then let it be. Who cares?

The size of my baby has more than doubled since the last ultrasound checkup. If I keep on feeding the child the way I have been, the baby would be approximately half of me at delivery. But that's not the truth.

So let´s eat.

YOUR BABY IS WHAT YOU EAT

From the first day of the official pregnancy confirmation by my favorite female doctor, I shifted my selfish thoughts right away from a mom-to-be to what´s the best for the baby. What to eat was not a challenge at first, because of my previous habits of preparing healthy meals and not eating junk food. Keeping the junk food under control should just be a breeze.

You can say that again, unless two buckets of your favorite ice cream just happen to be hidden in your freezer, and, all of a sudden, you discover them when you have no energy to cook dinner. OK, not a big deal. I will just have a few spoonfuls now and be done with it.

Did I say finish both buckets at the same time? I did.

Bread is going out of style, so everyone, please, just eat all you can now. After I put my hands on the two-pound bag, say good-bye to leftovers. The shape, size, or color of that bread or pastry doesn't matter, just as long as it was freshly baked this morning. I guarantee you that it will be eaten fresh today.

Let´s just assume for a second that, by some chance, there are some leftovers for tomorrow. Oh, in that case, you should not worry about any three-day-old bread. We (the baby and I) will definitely finish everything, and I mean every crumb of what´s leftover on the second day. Definitely there will be no three-day-old bread in the house.

Some women gain the same amount during an entire pregnancy as I did in the first three months.

HOT AND SOUR. WHAT´S YOUR FLAVOR?

My mom´s secret recipe to keep her face looking young and fresh is to clean it with a few drops of fresh lemon juice in the evening. I guess it's not a secret anymore, since I spelled it out here. Unfortunately I cannot prove her right or wrong, because my energy in the evening hours is just high enough to barely brush my teeth. So everything else is too much beatification.

One day I had more-than-enough energy to cut a small slice of lemon, but, before I had time to check in the mirror if my face was clean, I ate the whole lemon. My cravings for strong flavors had just started to produce those juices inside my mouth, and I was out of control.

My favorite foods were those with hot and sour flavors. The amount of hot was never spicy enough nor was the amount of sour ever tart enough. Most of the time I wasn't even hungry, but those pickles and their acidic brine water from the jar really kept me alive.

I purchased bigger jars of pickles now that would normally sit chilling in the fridge. There was also an extra jar "hidden" in a grocery bag at the bottom of my pantry, so that a few days later, if I had already eaten the extra jar from the pantry shelves and was left with only half or an almost empty jar in the fridge, I still had one more in reserve.

Balsamic vinegar took up most of my salad bowl, and it still didn't feel sour enough. More vinegar!

How about some sauerkraut on top of a pizza?

Ah, yeah, bring it, with extra sauerkraut and hot peppers.

For who-knows-what-reason, restaurants don't make those kinds of pizzas, so I had the luxury of indulging myself at home with a take-out pizza, made the way I like it. Really sour.

Good thing this was not a craving for sweets, and chocolate was not on my shopping list instead. My ass would have been bigger than that small country I was making fun of earlier.

OTHER ADDICTIONS AND PORTIONS SIZE

It seemed as if everyone had their own theory on guessing the gender of the baby, and I have also wondered if the baby's gender determines Mom's food cravings.

In my case, chocolate was not my craving when pregnant, luckily. Not to say that I couldn't finish a big box of chocolate in under one minute and feel good about it. If

I kept an inventory of all chocolates consumed in those nine months, it would really boil down to a few boxes of candy and whatever extra found on a few ice cream sticks.

Fruits and vegetables, on the other hand, were my addictions. The only difference now was that the portions were out of control. Give me two large salads now, and, if no one else was looking, I could eat a third one right away. Let´s not even mention that I had had three servings of fruit that morning, just one hour before we jumped into the brunch menu. I can´t blame the baby yet, because the baby can´t even defend himself.

At times I would pretend that I had no clue what´s going on and what kind of foods add up to just a bit over two thousand calories. One bowl of soup was never enough, so I had to eat one more bowl right afterward. There was always a justifiable thought that the baby needs it now, and the baby is growing, so I am eating healthy, eating for two. Two adults maybe.

Eating half of the XXXL-size water melon was OK, because it had a low calorie count. Not being able to stop after a few slices or after a stomachache is what I called out-of-control eating.

TWO WHEELS IS BETTER THAN FOUR WHEELS

It was the bicycle commute to work that kept the weight in a normal range during the first few months. Three miles to and three more back from work was a reasonable workout when added up for one week or a month. Then I moved to a different neighborhood, so the drive was reduced by a half. The food intake crept up slowly, doubling in no time.

It was uncomfortable to tie my shoes. While my hips were expanding, and my behind was getting bigger simultaneously, I was feeling out of shape. It was hard to tell if it was the baby or the fat on my belly that was also getting out of hand.

The first admission that I was overeating was harsh. If I keep up this pace, well, let´s just say that I can´t go on like that. I mean it. Literally. Wouldn't be able to walk so I can't continue like that.

The challenge of reducing my food intake to the same amount it had been before I was pregnant and only adding a few extra calories that the baby needed sounded easy. Supplementing with fruits and vegetables, and not with a double-size pasta plate before bedtime plus extra butter and cheese, sounded like a doable alternative.

Any excuse to make extralong trips on my bicycle was a good option. I felt lucky having no car, no four-wheeled vehicle, at the beginning of my second trimester.

I had no idea what it was like to gain weight so quickly, and I definitely didn't want to know what it will involve to take it off.

HOW OLD IS TOO YOUNG TO BE OLD?

I took one week of sick time during my first trimester due to my burned-out condition dealing with all the side effects my pregnancy brought me. Although I still felt weak after my sickation, I was not able to take another sick week later and juggle my work assignments. I couldn't find the appropriate time away from work. I didn't even have the energy to visit my doctor and ask for another week off.

Why am I losing my breath while talking? Is it that I am out of shape? No! It can't be. Am I really too old to be taking the stairs instead of an elevator to get to the fourth floor?

I wonder how much of a difference it would have made if I was pregnant while in my twenties or early thirties?

What gave me the most energy was the big smile from my doctor during each ultrasound, delivering nothing but good news. Baby was growing normally, and that's all I wanted to hear from her. She even made one comment that I have a talent at this age to make a perfect baby.

She would poke him around, and he would move and kick. On one occasion she waved at him while looking at the monitor and touching him again, and he waved back.

All the extra tests that were not covered by the insurance company, I gladly paid for them and whatever else she recommended in order to verify there was no risk associated with my age.

Another thing I appreciated about my pregnancy was the time of the year when I became pregnant, as far as what foods and vegetables were available. I was having cravings for cherries, because they were in season, as well as farmer's strawberries and other nonimported produce. Not only was I overbuying them but also overeating them by the buckets.

Plus the summer was not too hot in northern Germany, so I appreciated keeping the apartment cool and staying indoors on those hot days. There were only a few hot days of 99-plus-degree that lowered my appetite, but every day I ate and was able to keep the food down.

No matter how many comparison tables show what is a normal range for a woman's growth versus her baby's growth, in a short time period my buttons started to pop open and those jeans of mine were too tight. My biggest bra got small quick, because I had at least four extra pounds' worth of boobs in the first-T.

SECOND TRIMESTER

CRUISING ALTITUDE

MONTH 4 - SEPTEMBER

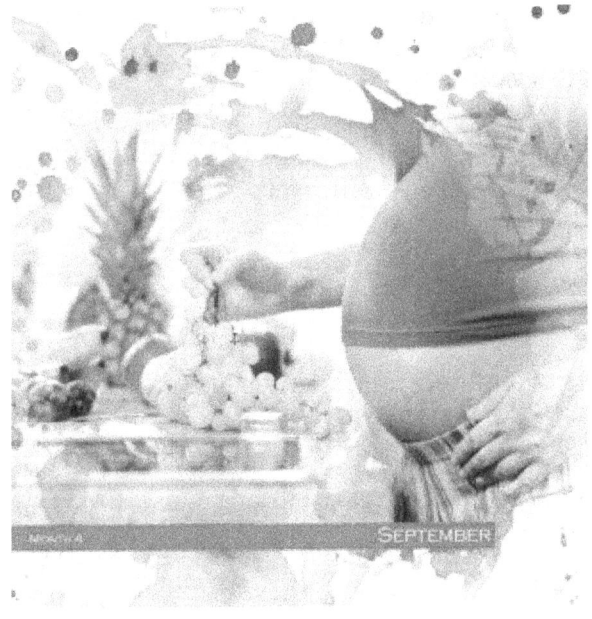

LITTLE (VAMPIRE) EMPIRE

I felt a sudden drop in energy around the same time each day. My interpretation was that the baby was feeding. This feeling would go away after about ten minutes, and, once I got used to it, I could plan that time for when I ate the energy-picker-upper foods.

Sometimes I would be busy or in the middle of a power nap during that time and may have missed the opportunity to fuel up with my energy-boosting foods. The way I would feel afterward was awful. A complete down-to-bottom, zero-energy feeling. Instantly I would know the cause of that energy depletion and that Baby was feeding while I was asleep.

Sucking the blood from another person is known to be done by vampires in fiction movies. Taking away energy from Mama was a baby trick that I had a hard time dealing with. I couldn't call the baby a little vampire, because we are talking about my baby now. No bad names please. No matter what.

Even when my energy before the nap would feel tall and strong, like the Empire State Building, yet after the nap would be at ground zero, still I can't blame the baby.

So that is how I came up with the baby nickname of a Little Empire.

My little prince that he is, he can't do anything bad to Mama.

I was the one who was supposed to educate myself about these things and take preventive actions.

My blood iron level dropped from 15.2 to 10.2 in seven months, and that was the reason I was feeling weak and looking pale late in my pregnancy. I was not prepared for this. I had it all firgured out wrong, including the shift for the daylight savings time event. At first I thought that this would be an advantage, since I could sleep one hour extra and be full of energy to go to work. In theory, yes, but in practice?

Moving the clock back one hour did have a big effect during the first few days, because I forgot that Baby will still feed at the same time as before. As I forgot the time shift, the baby would have a meal and drain my energy when I was not expecting it.

He was only doing what Mother Nature programmed him to do.

He did everything right.

A TO-DO LIST

I got advice from a friend based on his experience with the birth of his first son. His wife had a long to-do list of things she wanted to complete before the child was born.

Her intentions were to finish everything first and then deliver the baby.

It turned out that her delivery was well after the estimated due date, and the baby continued to grow now at a faster rate, causing concern. Could it be that she was the cause of the missed due date because of her unfinished to-do list?

I will not be prolonging my baby's birth deliberately because of unfinished housework, even if I knew how to do that. My own to-do list looked boring now compared to where it stood in my first trimester. The progress I made in the past months was visible, because the biggest item from my to-do list was scratched off. I had moved out of my smaller apartment in order to have a nursery. Boy, was I busy.

I had to arrange for someone to paint the apartment. After that I shopped for furniture, filling up all other empty spaces and corners with appliances and other necessary accessories which a new place needed. How much of a stress was that? Hard to tell because the process was long, so there were days of success and celebration and then days of small progress.

The feeling of *nesting* was kicking in, and finally I started feeling at home and ready for the little one.

WAS I REALLY LIKE THAT TOO?

Some things don't change in the second trimester, but the attitude toward pregnancy does, especially after observing another pregnant women. I am not as frantic as before about my constant visits to the potty room, food cravings, increase in weight, and shopping for larger clothes. I just accept it as it comes.

The pile of clothes I've put aside for a while is getting bigger and so what? Things that don't fit me will have to wait after childbirth for me to trim down my weight until I am able to wear my original clothes again.

The last day I wore normal jeans, the button was a bit of a stretch in a sitting position, so I changed the style to open-fly. After lunch, it didn't get any easier, so the pain in my waist was a good reminder to stock up on new clothes. I only had two pairs of pants now that would fit me.

Shopping that day was as expected, with poor results. Out of the three stores visited, I luckily found one equipped for mamas-to-be. The selection was small, and what was a good fit I was happy to take. I have now stocked up on all sizes for slim mama. After those things don't fit anymore, I will end up compromising in the large section for regular women's clothes with some XL numbers.

In the middle of my search for pants, one woman jumped in front of me, as if I was not there. I moved aside and went into another section, thinking, wow, she must be in her firsty (first trimester). Without paying too much attention to her, I walked away and got busy flipping through items and checking things out.

Now as I waited in line for a fitting room, guess who shows up behind me? The same woman. Politely I sized up her belly, and, sure enough, there was a bit of a baby bump, plus the child by her side must have been five to six years old. So she has some experience being pregnant.

I was wondering if I was also walking around like that, cutting people off, so loaded and ready to fire for no reason. My biting someone's head off doesn't look so bad now, when compared to this woman. I wasn't as aggressive, I think. For sure it was comforting, for a moment, to see someone else having a bad day and to think that my own was never that bad. I have handled my bad days better.

ONE CANNOT SEE SELF

I was the mirror image of the woman from the shopping event, I confess now. Only I don't walk around with a mirror the whole day long, so I cannot see myself. But that's not true.

What I can see are the faces of other people who had to deal with me. And that is if I was lucky and my hormones didn't blind me. Sometimes my closest friends and family were not there, because they used the exit strategy. All of a sudden they would have other business to do, so they could vanish as quickly as possible from my side.

On a few occasions I was even getting emotional, and it didn't feel so nice to be the one who people were avoiding. A few people needed a couple days off, while some pretended that I was bearable but still couldn´t wait for me to leave.

Can I blame them?

Not at all.

Maybe that is the reason I never mentioned anything to them and just played their game and supported their decision to be away from me. During those times alone, I´ve had a chance to look back and see my own mistakes.

Thanks, guys, for putting up with me, especially those who didn't even know I was pregnant.

WHY HAVE A BABY?

There is no right or wrong answer on why to have children.

What is your answer?

Different individuals have different answers. We are all different.

Some want to pass on their genes or to leave a legacy or to continue their family name.

Others may have a baby in order to change or obtain a new family name.

The view may be religious.

The list of reasons continues with endless combinations and options, so let me describe my own.

For decades I have had more reasons why not to have kids than to have them. There were times I didn't want kids, because I didn't think I could afford them. There were periods when I was so busy and had no time to have kids. Sometimes it did not matter if my family line ended or continued.

There were times when I was with the wrong partner or lived some place not ideal for raising a family. There were times when I wasn't sure and was waiting to be sure. Then I would change my mind from wanting to not wanting in a matter of seconds and back to who-knows-which-choice and at which time.

The first time I felt strongly about having kids was while learning karate and having the opportunity to help my sensei in the children's class. Can there be anything cuter than watching these young students meditate at the beginning and end of each session? Maybe I felt a strong bond with them because we were on the same level, as I was learning how to meditate too.

Why have a baby? I had to meditate on that for months and months to come.

HOW MANY WEEKS LEFT?

One thing that got on my nerves during the first half of my pregnancy was this weekly count, and my doctor´s reference to week X or XX. Dividing the pregnancy into trimesters was a better alternative for me, since it came as a relief to know that one-third of my pregnancy journey was over.

Or to think that I am halfway there was a good feeling of accomplishment. Of course I want to forget all my misery and have something to look forward to.

The second half.

Doesn't that sound much better than, uhm, let´s see? Was that week seventeen, eighteen, or nineteen? Do I start the new week now? Well, I can´t quite figure it out.

Another twenty weeks to go or what?

Four months and two weeks. Oh, yeah, Baby, that sounds good, because nine months divided by two, that even sounds better than that I am in a first week of my second trimester.

Is that by the Gregorian or lunar calendar?

What? Come again!

Why make this more complicated than it is already?

At some point I got a bit confused and counted those damn weeks incorrectly, so I celebrated my halfway mark too early. At the end somehow it still felt as if there wasn't much left.

So far I had carried this little one for four and a half months and took the best care I could of this precious baby inside me. And I did not fall off my bicycle or fall off my chair while taking a nap in the office. I did not lift anything too heavy that caused internal bleeding. To the best of my knowledge, I have not caused any pain to this child.

MONTH 5 - OCTOBER

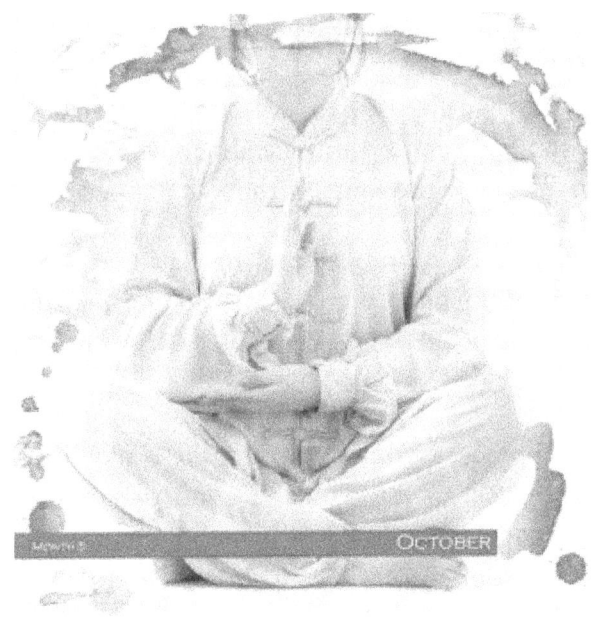

HALFTIME

I am not yet ready to look ahead, since I am too busy celebrating the end of the first half of my pregnancy. Friends are already trying to scare me with the stories of how the last part of the pregnancy will be the most difficult.

I am counting on Mother Nature to do her part, just the way she is supposed to, so there is no need for me to worry about some things right now. Let the things happen when it is the time for them to happen.

I am not the only one celebrating halftime. Thanks to the father of the baby, who has played an important part in the child's healthy development, we are enjoying this milestone together.

He contributed, not only by lifting the heavy things that would have been a bit too much for me to carry alone, but by carrying an invisible load—by not giving me any extra stress. He understood when the hormones of a pregnant woman were talking and not a reasonable human being.

And that's all there is to it. Pregnancy can produce an unreasonable, demanding, highly explosive person, just ready to blow out something nasty.

WHAT A DREAM

Yesterday morning I had a dream about my baby. The dream happened quickly, so I remembered only a few details, but I did not see his face, which was very interesting to me.

In one part of the dream he was lying on the stairs, and that made me very upset, because he was in danger of falling down. So I was giving my sister and my cousin a hard time for leaving him there and not watching him.

The weird part of the dream, which I did not like at all, was that he was born prematurely and that I was only able to hold him for a while before he had to go back (you know where). At first, I was breast-feeding, and then I picked him up, facing me, so he could stand on my knees.

At that time he started to laugh and grabbed me by the shoulders with his two small arms. I felt his firm grip and strength, which made me very proud. Then he put his face on mine gently, somewhere around my nose and cheek area, as if he would suck on my face or kiss it. And I just laughed.

The best part of the dream was that, after telling my boyfriend of this, I had tears in my eyes.

That was the dream, and, as with most of my dreams, I never knew what to make of them. Sometimes, if it was a bad dream, I could say, OK, be careful at work or while traveling or something like that, but, most of the time, I just forgot about them, and nothing happened afterward.

If I had to make some sense out of this dream, it was to not let my sister watch my child. Oh, my gosh, that was so rude to say, but let's continue with the story. The other part was not to worry myself to death about not being able to breast-feed and people giving formula to my kid, because all that extra worry could maybe lead into an early delivery of a premature baby, and then I would really be stuck with this dream.

And don't forget the best part of the dream: he was a very strong child, happily smiling and giving Mama kisses on the face, and I was breast-feeding him. Don't forget that the child never let me see his face in the dream, and I never saw any kind of clothing that would conclude the sex of the baby.

Just like in reality, sometimes the ultrasound can be faulty, and babies predicted to be boys turn out to be girls at birth, so I should also accept the fact that Baby is a baby, no matter what, and I should not be biased.

TO MEAT OR NOT TO MEAT

For more than a decade now I do not eat things that have at least two feet. The most common answer I give for why I do this is:

"I just don't crave it anymore."

I want to say much more, but this is the quickest way to get people off my back. If the person is not satisfied with my answer and persists with additional questions, sometimes I would add:

"If I ever got pregnant, and I had a craving to eat sausage or fried chicken or anything of that sort, I would start eating meat again. But not until then."

My mom told me an interesting story from the time she was pregnant with me. In the first trimester she had morning sickness, and, among the many things that made her sick to her stomach, the one that made her vomit the most was the smell of meat cooking.

I have to admit that, 99 percent of the time before my pregnancy, to me also meat cooking smelled yucky, but, 1 percent of time, the only type of meat preparation that did not bother me was barbecue. Maybe because the smoke was blocking the actual smell, but really that was the only time I could ignore it, but not all the time.

Now during my pregnancy, not only the smell of cooking meat stinks to me but it would put me in a bad mood too. Me, in a bad mood? What an excuse to justify my temper.

Seriously, even as a guest, I would tell people how their kitchen smelled to me and that they should open up the kitchen windows but close the kitchen doors, so the odor does not spread around the house. Just think how welcome I was after that visit, but I didn't care.

Beef was the worst smell for me, while cooking. It really could make me scream. One of my hosts was preparing a soup that not only contained beef but two additional meats, which I am even afraid to mention. When you mix up three dead animals in one pot, trust me when I say a different beast comes out of it.

This story was not supposed to give people who eat meat a hard time, because, I swear, I would have no friends or family left to talk to if I was discriminating against their own diet choices. Just like with everything else, everyone can live their life the way they want to and make their own decisions about what's good for them or not.

However, I do have a choice of what to feed my own kid in the first few years. Later this child will be exposed in kindergarten to all kinds of meat products. Simply while hanging out with his daddy, the kid will get a taste of meat. So no need for me to fuss and scream, because, most likely, I will lose this battle.

I asked my boyfriend that, before he offers meat to the child, can he take the kid to someone's farm first and show what the animal looks like alive?

So let me not pretend to be an angel (technically I am a lacto ovo vegetarian) and finally confess.

In the second trimester I ate fish. It was a hot, spicy fish soup that my boyfriend had prepared for me on my birthday. I had forgotten that the main ingredient was fish. To me, the pot was full of love, and that's all that mattered.

GOT MILK?

I stopped drinking cow's milk more than twenty years ago, and that was way before I even knew anything about the vegan/vegetarian lifestyle. My choice at that time was for a different reason. I had moved from Europe to the States, and the taste of milk was like day and night. To me it had some funny taste to it, which I cannot even describe up to this day. Plastic? Maybe from the milk carton or the gallon container?

If I won't drink cow's milk, I sure don't want my son drinking it. What if for some reason I am not able to breast-feed?

The last choice in the world to feed my baby is the baby formula based on cow's milk as a substitute for my own milk. Cow's milk is for baby cows and not for baby humans. Cows are a totally different species.

I don't even want to use the "green" excuse and let's save the planet as an issue here. I don't want to mention anything about the dairy industries.

I just want to figure out what to feed my child in case I am unable to breast-feed, for whatever reason.

Soy milk baby formula is not an option, and I am not happy about any of the choices right now offered in the grocery stores.

I have spent days and days researching this subject, and I have visited sites from different governments, pages in countries with known religions that are not consuming milk, and read blogs by other experienced moms. I have also read published scientific research papers, and not only was I exhausted from my search but I was even more worried, to the point that I almost want to give up and give damn formula to my child.

How sad that is. The more I read about baby formulas, the more I wanted to stay away from them, yet there wasn't a good alternative to breast-feeding.

C'mon. Why am I so stubborn?

Why am I horrified of the two o'clock in the morning baby-feeding time?

I can just add hot water to this wonder powder and watch my baby grow.

I wish.

I went back to square one and spent hours reading about breast-feeding. I felt a little better as I was building more hope for the best possible solution.

WASHING FRUITS

It was important to me to learn simple things I can do during my pregnancy to prevent stupid things from happening. For example, to wash all my fruits and vegetables thoroughly before eating them, so I don't end up in the hospital.

Wow, slow down. How did I end up there so quick?

Is paranoia also one of the side effects during pregnancy? Not that I am aware of.

It is not the dirt that scares me or some soil leftover on my carrot. It is the chemicals they use to wash that carrot before it is packaged or the pesticide used to grow that carrot that I am troubled with. If I was too paranoid, then I would never eat anything, so let's be ignorant for a while and assume the carrot was grown naturally, without added chemical help.

When I grow that carrot, and harvesttime comes, I will just pull it out of the ground, wash the dirt off with some cold water and bite into it. Unfortunately my garden is still under development in my head, so the carrot that I get is from a grocery store.

Who and what touched that carrot is what makes me fearful. The contamination from people's dirty hands is the worst thing on my mind. The grocery cart handle is a nasty environment, so the customers can contaminate the entire store, plus the workers who put the carrot on display, and the cashier touching it again, not to mention the loading and unloading by more people in the transport of the food from farm to market.

There are plenty of places for that carrot to contact things—surfaces and places that were already in some ways dirty and full of germs.

If I make a mistake and forget to wash that carrot, then I end up consuming some horrible thing from polluted hands and/or places.

And?

And the list of toxins can go on forever.

At minimum I end up with diarrhea.

Dehydration.

Mama not eating.

Baby not eating.

Maybe that is how Mama ends up in the hospital and all from what?

A dirty carrot.

THE HIPS AND THE PAIN NOT SO HIP

It doesn't matter how many different names you give to a pregnant woman, she still remains a pregnant woman. Maybe grouchy, cranky, and jumpy too.

Why?

The list of things that bother her goes on, but no one seems to care.

That's why.

For example, let's talk about the hips of a pregnant woman.

Pregnant women experience cramps and pains in their

hips, and one cannot even describe how much pain there is. The pain could be there after she gets up in the morning or after sitting for a while or after lying down. So there is this pain that she just ends up dealing with and ignoring most of the time. It feels as if her whole body is falling apart, because the area is inundated with the pain.

Am I appreciating this pain because it means that my body is getting ready to make room for the baby, to have enough space so it can pass through?

I am not thinking that way. I am thinking, now why in the world is this hurting so much?

When I walk, I can feel so stiff that I can't even tell anymore if walking is helping or making things worse. I take small steps, focusing on my posture, the center of gravity, and my weight distribution. I mean, c'mon, that's a lot of engineering going on during a walk.

We can only get used to it, and that's all there is to it.

No pain, no gain.

FROM BACK PAIN TO NO BACK PAIN WITH A LITTLE BIT OF TWO CHINESE MARTIAL ARTS

I started getting lower back pain again, which I hadn't suffered with in years. The pregnancy was not so much to blame as was my increase in weight, plus a combination of previous issues and a sucky contribution. Having an office job and sitting most of the time inappropriately for the past seventeen years was the sucky contribution part. Previous issues go back to my childhood, having a little kyphosis (a rounded upper back) and extreme textbook-example scoliosis (lateral curvature of the spine).

Well, if you do the math correctly, these two issues can also cause headaches and make a person tired.

How do I know?

I had to do the dirty work and figure out the cause of the pain on my own, because not a single doctor could find the reason.

As many people have troubles with back pains, most of the time the cause is the hardest to identify. What most people end up with are multiple screening tests and doctors' experiments with treatments, such as heating pads, massages, and physical therapy sessions. Discouragement or, in extreme cases, a nervous breakdown on top of the back pain is a well-known side effect for those suffering patients who can identify no cause for their pain.

About twelve years ago I learned tai chi, so that did it for me. It got rid of the back pain. First the headaches disappeared slowly, then the back pain. A few years later one of my masseuses said that she had never seen anyone's spine go through as much positive change in such a short period of time. It was a miracle.

If you have a good Tai Chi Master, you will be learning a little about qi gong too, and so did I. After years of practice, I ended up actually enjoying these arts. It is still somewhat mechanical more than intuitive for me, so I wouldn't brag about my abilities. Let's just say that I have know-how.

My routine starts in the morning before work. I meditate and perform tai chi movements. No matter what time, and no matter how late I may be for work, I still end up spending at least twenty minutes in my routine. Before you start to believe that I am a disciplined individual, then let me assure you that I am not. Because doing tai chi twice a day has not yet become a habit. I can do well for weeks and months, and yet slip again to only morning sessions.

My tiredness and achy body left me with no option but to turn my attempt at well-being to Eastern practices instead of Western (visits to the doctors).

The lower back pain started to kick in early in the evening. Cooking dinner and standing by the stove or washing the dishes was too much now. My patience was wearing thin, and this time there was no one to blame. I had to do something about it. So I changed the way I stand.

I was now doing a horse-stance instead of just balancing on my two feet. Those lunch hours, when I used to look for a place to take a quick nap, were now replaced with ten-minute qi gong sessions. I saw benefits in less than one week.

The best part about all this was bonding with the baby, building my flexibility and strength. I am also more aware of my balance, because I know when I perform certain tai chi steps now that I am pregnant, I lose my balance more frequently. That extra weight can throw me off, so I adjust. I need to take smaller steps and slow down a bit while doing any normal thing (walking, bending down, etc.).

NOT A DULL MOMENT

After reaching halftime, Baby's kicks and movements were more frequent and active, so I never felt alone. The anticipation of his kicks was exciting. Maybe the next move would be a new maneuver that I had not felt before.

When he was the size of a banana, on one occasion I had a feeling that he did a complete 180-degree turn, or maybe a double salto, plus one more flip, or whatever trick he was pulling in there. I did not have a good idea of how much room he had to play in, or what his arms and legs were capable of doing, so it was a wonderful guessing game.

Being pregnant didn't seem that hard after all in the second trimester, and even the thoughts of having a second child were crossing my mind, from all the special joy of having this little one making me feel so special.

HAPPY MAMA-TO-BE, AND HAPPY TO BE MAMA

They say that a mind can have as many as 64,000 thoughts

in one day. During my pregnancy, half those thoughts were almost certainly baby-related.

On any day the anxiety could be experienced on one level and then change another day to a different level. Fear is fear. The fear of certain events or the fear of things that will probably never happen, yes, they too also cross a woman´s mind during pregnancy.

I would be embarrassed if some of my fears were recorded and replayed later. They were foolish and unnecessary, but they still took place. The unknown was always at the top of the list when it came to fear, and then, when mixed with another unknown factor, it was easy to guess my state of happiness.

If I came across as rude, jumpy, angry, and not so pleasant to be around, it´s because of those 64,000 thoughts that I had on my mind.

This changed later, and the amount of my happiness increased as the baby grew. Baby´s father was also around more, and, with that, the amount of laughs in my days increased.

As the days were passing by, I was a happier mama-to-be.

HOW MUCH FREEDOM WILL THE CHILD HAVE?

I think totally opposite from an average parent.

Why?

Maybe because I am not a parent yet.

It never crossed my mind to push the child to become a doctor or a lawyer, engineer, a dentist, or whatever our parents wished from us back in those days when the character of the person was judged by a title and the name of the institution from where the title was obtained.

Does that mean that I would discourage my child from pursuing one of those careers? Not exactly but I would not push it to the point that my child ends up hating everything about his childhood.

Similar with sports. Some people overdo it with the baseball, soccer games, driving kids two hours to the practice location and getting them back home after 10:00 p.m. That's the type of parent I will try not to be. Instead I will support the love and talent my child has and encourage him to be as good at it as he can, without overdoing it.

So how to find that perfect balance?

No way of knowing now. I just have to wait and see.

RUNNING OUT OF TIME - IT'S ACTION TIME

It seemed as if it was just yesterday that I was still in my first trimester.

Why is the time running faster now?

Is it?

How come it seems so soon?

At first a vaginal birth sounded good. It is time to do this part right, right?

What about the alternative?

What if I have no choice?

The complications may be there, regardless of the choice, together with the pain.

So we are going with a vaginal birth, right?

Are you sure?

How long before I change my mind and think the other way?

Vaginal seemed longer and more painful when compared to a C-section. The scary statistics for vaginal labor talk about lasting twenty-four to thirty hours. On the other hand, the aftermath has a very positive side compared to a C-section. Taking a shower, sneezing, sitting or bending down, all of those activities should be easier to perform after a vaginal birth.

We are going vaginal.

Which one is correct? How should it be, and what law determines my baby's nationality and citizenship?

A German is anyone born in Germany.

A German has a German father.

Baby's mother is a German.

Born in Germany and one of the parents is German.

Born in Germany and both parents are German.

German parent is also a born German or a naturalized German.

Yes, it gets complicated.

My choice of nationality, if I had one, would be who-knows-what. I was married before to a naturalized American, and his parents were also not born there. So that makes me a perfect American.

Not really.

My baby will be German, because it will be born in Germany, and the father is a naturalized German. My baby will also be American because of his right for a dual citizenship and my own status. So go figure.

Which language will my baby be learning?

He better not learn German from me, because I planned to learn German from and with the baby. It is better not to learn English from me, because I have not mastered it either, and that's after twenty years of living in an English-speaking country.

MY NIPPLES. NOW WHY?

Come on, moms. You all have had kids and know what will happen, so why are you keeping quiet?

How many times did you tell someone bluntly:

"Sit your ass down and let me tell you about all the things you will go through."

Why do I have to wake up one day and look at my dark nipples, but I have no clue why they are like dark chocolate? And what am I supposed to do now? Call the doctor, or jump on the Internet and do a search?

Empress, I am tired of looking up everything on the Web. Why? Because so many things are normal during pregnancy, and I can spend hours and hours learning about one condition, until another normal condition shows up. Why didn't anyone tell us about these things before we got pregnant? Maybe we would think twice about getting pregnant.

Scaring teenagers not to get pregnant is a different lesson. But, once you are pregnant, you are really screwed, because you are still on your own. Your mother, sister, cousin, and friend will tell you everything that is less important than what you really end up experiencing on your own. It doesn't really have to be that way.

As a grown-ass woman, I should know all about it. Bitches and queens, stop hiding the truth and start telling every little thing to everyone. Things you have suffered with.

Go on Oprah's show, for God's sake.

Most of the celebrities who end up telling stories about having kids make it look so easy, and only a few tell the truth. I know you will tell me the other half of the truth: that women have been doing this now since the beginning of time.

My grandma raised seven kids, and she never made a fuss about it, I am sure some smart-ass will say. She had to take care of the land and all the farm animals, and she did fine.

Well, smarty-pants, how the heck do you know that she did fine? Did anyone ever ask her how she was doing?

HOW TO INTERPRET BABY KICKS AND MOVES

Besides thinking of my baby as a gymnast, I, at times, interpreted his talents as moods he was going through. Sometimes, when I laugh out loud, after about a ten-second delay, he would definitely turn around.

The same thing would happen at dinnertime. About one

minute after I start eating, the baby would also start to turn around, so I would interpret that as him being happy. If I was in bed laying down sideways and pushing a bit on my stomach, I would interpret his moves as if he did not have enough room to move around, so now he is kicking me back.

There were times when I would feel small and fast vibrations in one spot or some movement in my kidney area, and those I did not know how to interpret. Regardless of what was going on and what those moves really meant, it didn't matter to me. I knew they were good things, and the baby was growing.

A few times I had a feeling that he found something in my stomach to kick—my liver, gallbladder, something he got creative with. Another time the feeling was as if he was pulling on his umbilical cord, like in small jerks. How long that cord is, I have no clue, but I also had a feeling that he was sideways bungee-jumping.

At times his moves kind of scared me, until I got used to it. Lying in the dark, you're half asleep, when, all of a sudden, something moves inside your stomach, and you don't know what moved. Then I knew that it´s the baby and that everything is all right.

Probably I have also freaked out the baby as much as he freaked me out. Sometimes the body makes funny noises. My stomach may be digesting something out loud, or I am passing some gas.

What was that, Mama? Not again.

HUNGER VERSUS CRAVINGS

As a tall person, I have the luxury of being able to gain weight without anyone noticing a few extra pounds. The first place for fat storage was in my stomach area, and my six-pack would lose a few packs. Now with the belly bump, I have no clue how much of that was fat and how much was a good thing to have.

Things were getting out of hand when I noticed a little fat area under my chin. I knew it was not a normal baby-weight gain, but it actually had a lot to do with my eating habits. What contributed to this issue was my midnight snacks, if one could even call them that. It was not at midnight first of all, and it could have been any time after midnight and before six in the morning. It was not always snack size either, more of an entire meal.

I was wide awake because of the potty business or things on my mind related to childbirth. So what choice do I really have? To drink water so my stomach feels full would only mean more trips to the bathroom.

To eat something that would knock me off the ground until I passed out sounded much better. Bananas had this effect on me. Somehow I only had the large ones in the house during my pregnancy. Sometimes eating a banana worked, and sometimes I was still up for a while.

What almost always worked was to have an omelet with three eggs. Usually they were smaller-than-average eggs, like that matters anyways, because the difference could be twenty to thirty calories, which is small compared to my total caloric intake. But this worked.

It usually got me *sooo* sleepy so quickly that I would forget to even count the calories for the bread with that meal. I was sound asleep, and that´s all that mattered to me. The temporary gratification of getting that sleep was more important than the calorie count.

Until …

Until a tall person started looking huge and there was no doubt that this person was pregnant but also couldn't control her food intake. There is a huge difference between eating when hungry and eating when bored or having cravings, and there is a price to pay for that.

The first price to pay is now, being aware of that extra weight. Later I am sure there will be a rude awakening, when the baby is borne, but the fat stays with me, as if I am still expecting a baby.

Am I saying good-bye to my six-pack forever? Well, not really. I am sure my body will remember being skinny and in shape most of my life, so I should bounce back quickly, because the muscles will remember how to tone down in no time.

I will be somewhat disappointed to see myself looking out of shape like never before after giving birth, but obviously that is only temporarily. I have other things on my mind right now. It's all about the well-being of the baby.

Probably the little one is also storing and consuming fat

in those small baby muscles, so we'll have to put him on a baby treadmill before he can even walk.

We'll invent a treadmill for crawling.

SECOND ULTRASOUND AND 3-D PHOTO

My boyfriend was present for our five-month ultrasound. The doctor asked if we wanted to know whether the child was a boy or a girl. I did not hear the question correctly and only heard the girl part.

"No," I yelled.

"Boy," the doctor said without even waiting on both of our answers.

I looked up at my boyfriend, and now he had more than a big smile on his face.

The best part of the second ultrasound was the confirmation again that the baby was normal. We could see his hands and five fingers on each, and we got a photo of his footprint.

I also learned where the baby's head was resting, so I could better interpret the different kicks in my stomach. The baby also smiled at one point, and the doctor was quick enough to catch that moment and give us that photo.

In the collection of photos, now we had Baby's profile,

one picture of him smiling, one baby footprint, and one picture of the baby's sex organ. The last photo was of his face in 3-D technology. This 3-D photo looked like a picture of a baby doll.

"He has his father's nose," explained the doctor.

"He has his father's lips," I exclaimed.

His cheeks too, which made him look really cute, because his face looked more round and full. My boyfriend also noticed that the baby's forehead was a spitting image of his own.

"How can it be that he has everything of yours?" I said with a smile on my face.

Later, while we were driving home, I projected my baby boy into the future and pictured him in his teen years. Since he will be good-looking, the first thing that crossed my mind was that some girl will be kissing those lips. Them little bitches will be kissing my boy.

"What?" asked my boyfriend.

"Yeah, those girls will be kissing my boy."

Later that night, while trying to fall asleep, the only image in my head was that color 3-D photo from the ultrasound. I had checked it out about one hundred times and then took a picture of that picture so I can have it saved on my phone. His image in my head also gave me extra strength to get up the next day and go to work.

Only for a few moments I wondered if the new 3-D

technology took something good out of this anticipation of having a child. I have to wait four more months before the baby arrives, but I already know what he looks like. So my answer was no, and I was happy to have this image in my head.

HOLDING A BABY

Yesterday my boyfriend and I visited one of his friends and his wife, who delivered a beautiful baby girl last month. It was a most precious experience for me, while pregnant, to hold another baby.

The baby girl was very quiet and happy. When she was tired, she yawned; when she was hungry, she cried; and the rest of the time, she was catching quick naps or looking around, curious as to who was this new woman now holding her. And while she may find me interesting to look at, she knows I am not her mama.

It is amazing how much a person can grow just by holding a baby. I have realized that, only now, after holding so many babies in my lifetime, almost none of those times had a full impact on me. It is only now, when I am expecting my own, that I have grown from a young lady to a woman.

They say that it takes a whole village to raise a child. Finally I am beginning to understand the real meaning of that saying, although I had already known what it meant. If I reverse that saying and instead write:

It takes a whole child to raise a village, it also has a nice meaning to it. Or how about:

It takes a small child to raise a woman.

STOPPED COUNTING AT CRUISING ALTITUDE

I still can't wait to see my newborn baby boy, but I have stopped counting the weeks and days.

Why?

If I am to compare it to the time spent at work on Friday afternoon, it is relatively the same, because time does not move on that clock. All other highly anticipated events of happiness are usually impacted by this funny time effect. The moment one forgets about it or gets distracted with other thoughts is when things usually start to happen faster.

A friend of mine has referenced one doctor´s statement describing pregnancy as an airplane trip. The first trimester is a period of takeoff, a little bit of a bumpy ride, with all kinds of mixed feelings of doubt. The second trimester is like cruising at high altitude without any turbulence. The third trimester is just like landing.

Right now I am enjoying cruising at the high altitude.

BABY DAYDREAMING AT WORK

During meetings at work, Baby would kick, and I couldn't help myself but laugh. He did his flips and turns, while I am the only one aware of it, and the other meeting participants have no clue of what's going on inside my stomach.

Of course I would try to communicate with him, let him know I am here, because maybe he feels alone and hasn't heard Mama's voice in a while. I would rub my stomach to see if he would kick back in the same spot where I rubbed.

Of course I am looking for any excuse to get distracted from work and to think about the baby. Sometimes I wonder what he may be dreaming of. Maybe nothing now but maybe he does have his own baby dreams.

Just like we can dream of places we have never been to and people we have never met, the baby too probably has dreams. I wonder what is in his pictures, when he has not seen the outside world yet.

Recently I read *Physics of the Future* by Michio Kaku, who writes about current technologies giving us the possibility to record dreams. Probably future ultrasounds will also have a built-in feature showing the baby's dreams.

All from the comfort of our living rooms.

I wish that technology was available now.

WHAT YOU EAT IS WHAT IT IS

There were times when I have had no control over what to eat, how much, and when. I wonder if that has something to do with the pregnancy hormones too, because usually I have pretty good control in that area. I have even given a new definition to brunch. I think it used to be the only meal somewhere in between breakfast and lunch. On my daily menu was breakfast, brunch, and lunch.

The order in which I have eaten the food that is usually assigned to each meal was also all backward. I could eat lunch for breakfast and breakfast for lunch; it did not matter at all. Sometimes just looking at the food gave me a craving to eat it right away, and it did not matter in which meal it belonged or what time of the day it was.

Only by the end of the second trimester could I consume only what was recommended, not overeat in the evening or before bedtime, or eat the appropriate meal for that time of the day. I have also noticed that, earlier in my pregnancy, buying a new bra stayed on the shopping list. They were getting smaller and smaller after each wash, and it was not because of the water or detergent I was using.

Each week a new pair of jeans was making the way into the area of my closet called To Be Worn Next Year. The pair that barely fit in the morning was already tight by brunch time, and I would be lucky if a scarf or a sweater could camouflage the belly area, so I could keep my pants unzipped and unbuttoned.

Even the pants with this funny extension designed for pregnancy, what I call *the pouch for the stomach*, can also be tight sometimes. Every now and then I would look at myself in the mirror and laugh because of the shape of my profile.

I really look like a kangaroo.

BELLY SIZE AND THE BODY PROFILE

In my first trimester, if I was lying on my back, my stomach was actually a big valley. It was only at the beginning of the fourth month that a little bump started to show. This was mainly due to my excessive eating during that time.

As my boobs were growing at a rapid speed in my first trimester, I would call a shopping day "good" if I could find three sizes of bras bigger than the one I was wearing that day. That would save me trips to the store in the next month at least.

But approaching the end of the fifth month, my body started to change again differently. My boobs were not growing exponentially any longer, and, for some reason, they were not as sensitive as before. I was not about to scream every time my boyfriend touched them. Or about to bite his head off. OK, maybe ready to bite his hand off.

What became more sensitive was my belly and the pain associated with small touches. Now it was my stomach that was getting in the way—and in a good way, I mean.

At some point my boyfriend's knuckles brushed my stomach, and I was furious.

I feel lucky that he has the patience to put up with me. No other man would keep up with my nasty self, pregnant or not. No excuses.

My body's profile had changed, so instead of my boobs sticking out the most, now my stomach did.

I could still see my toes over my nose.

☺

Ha, ha. No wait. I mean, over my stomach.

But there was one part of my body that was now hidden, under my stomach, and it was becoming more and more difficult to maintain that "lawn." Of course I could have my boyfriend be the gardener, but we all know where that would lead. … Straight into the bedroom.

To keep it all bushy was not an option.

That lawn needs a makeover.

MONTH 6 - NOVEMBER

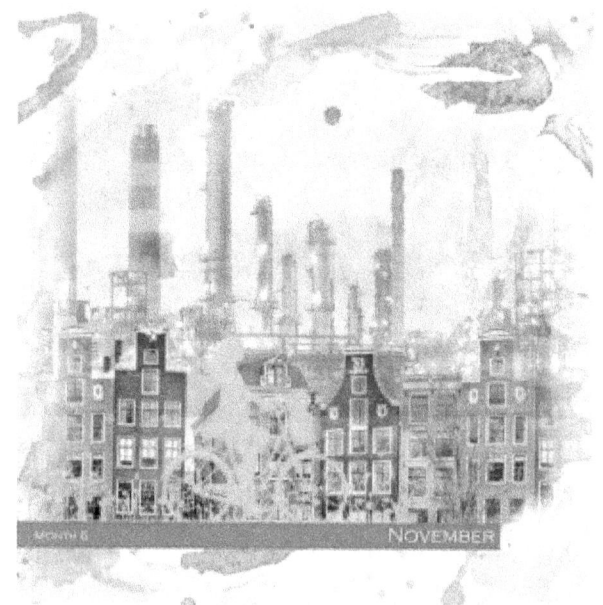

DON'T TELL ME WHAT'S NORMAL

In the second trimester I had less desire to read about the weekly progress for pregnancies and what is considered a "normal" experience.

Why?

It started to irritate and annoy me.

Ignorance is bliss sometimes, and knowledge can be really useless in this case.

Why do I need to know that an increase in vaginal discharge is normal?

What can I do about it?

The clitoris is extrasensitive. Whoop-de-do.

Multiple orgasms are also normal during this time. I´ll take those as they come, but I wouldn't fuss about it if they don't.

Why stress about it?

That´s normal.

PUT UP AND SHUT UP

My weight is increasing, is on the rise, and I have a good justification in order not to flip out and feel overweight.

I think for every 100 grams (3.5 ounces) that Baby gained, I ended up also gaining close to one kg (2.2 pounds). So right now he is 966 grams or close to two pounds. You can do the math as to how much I have gained.

Here is my estimated calculation of where the weight went. Please keep in mind these are not technical or medical terms.

Tits, about three kilos (6.6 pounds).

Ass, an extra two kilos (4.4 pounds).

In my hips, there are probably two more kilos (4.4 pounds).

In my face/chin about half a kilo (about 1 pound).

I am typing right now with my mouthful of food, so a few hundred grams (less than 1 pound) are there.

HIGHS AND LOWS

I have to use this comparison now, as I transition from my second to third trimester. The energy just changed from high to a low in less than two seconds. It is a real roller-coaster ride. Except there was not even enough energy left in me to scream while coming down. I just dropped. No special announcements, just feeling blah.

Maybe that glucose test today had a lot to do with it. First I had the big breakfast, which was recommended by the doctor's nurse. Then I had to bike a decent distance in a rush to make it to my 9:00 a.m. appointment. To drink that sugary cold water took some effort on my part, because I am not used to drinking sweet beverages or cold ones.

While sugar-high, I had to lay still, so they could measure my labor contractions for twenty minutes. Then they rushed me to the examination room for my doctor to check out things. Back in the lab for more blood tests. In the meantime, the nurse discovered that they were supposed to run one more blood test a while back, which meant drawing more blood.

By the time all the tests were completed, it was almost lunchtime, so I stopped by the house and ate a little more before heading to work. Now I bike the additional miles to work, so, in total, the exercise amount added up to a decent number for that morning. As I arrived in my office, I started to crash.

Working for the rest of the day was no fun at all, except that my office mate went on a business trip that afternoon, and my inbox was empty, so I could plan my workday the way I wanted it. That helped a little.

Not wearing any makeup that day added the extratired

look to my face. That´s to be polite and to not say that I looked like hell. By the time I had biked back home after work, the tiredness started to really kick in. Now this is the time when the hunger is persistent, but I have no energy to make a meal or warm up any leftovers. Dirty dishes from breakfast and lunch can be dirty as they want to be, and the sink may be calling for some attention, but there is no force that could make me do anything about it at that moment.

The only option is to lie down and try to sleep. Hard to sleep when the hunger is kicking in. The baby is tired too.

How long I was quiet and not moving on the couch, I am not sure. It was time to refuel. These are the times when I also appreciate being a health freak and having all those energy-boosting foods in my house.

I had a fresh coconut, so I drank a glass of coconut water first. Then I chopped my power vegetables into a medium-size bowl. There was no need to add millions of things when it was wiser to prepare it as soon as possible and eat it right away. I had one beet, a handful of fresh spinach, broccoli, and the meat from that fresh coconut. My meal tasted as if there were hundreds of ingredients, and nothing was missing. Halfway through the salad, I was already feeling 100 percent better.

Replacing all that blood loss took at least one more day. One salad cannot replace it all, and I required more eating, drinking, and sleeping to feel somewhat stronger. The baby also kept quiet during this time. Only when I felt his strong pulls on the umbilical cord the next day did I know he was all right and that Mama was doing fine too.

WORK IS HAZARDOUS TO MY HEALTH

The production of chemicals is a strictly regulated business, and there are laws to protect each employee where chemicals are produced. One of those laws is to know what hazards are present and if there are special personal protective measures that need to be in place to prevent the personnel from exposures. Occasionally I am required to walk in the heart of the chemical plant, inside the control rooms, or to walk from one building to another while passing close by the production site.

For a jumbo company located on a large chemical site that is shared with other chemical giants, the amount of chemicals present can easily be in the tens of thousands. For me, the concern was getting exposed to any of the substances that are colorless and odorless and harmful in small quantities, without me even knowing about it.

If that's not nasty enough, the measuring devices used to detect those substances, such as radioactive gadgets, or X-ray equipment, can also be hazardous and risky for pregnant women. My baby is not yet fully developed or strong, and I may walk through fumes that may contain cancer-causing chemicals.

I have no choice but to work under those conditions. Maybe the only hazard was my own stress level about the hazards, and there was no damage whatsoever.

I hope.

SLEEP HOURS

My sleep patterns were as upside down as they could be, or should I call them sleepless patterns? The baby was getting stronger, and my energy was dropping aggressively in the evening hours after work. Due to daylight savings time, I could not stay awake to 10:00 p.m. any longer, and even waiting for 8:30 p.m. took a lot of effort on my part.

A good night's sleep meant getting up only about five times and not being awake for hours in the bed. I have had days when I was in bed before nine, was lucky to sleep a total of eight (interrupted) hours, and would be asleep at eight in the morning, only to rush out of bed to not be late for work. Sometimes rushing out of bed was not as important as calling in late. Not showing up to work was not as difficult as it once was. I had no shame to say, "I have overslept, and I didn't sleep well," or that "I am not coming to work at all."

Since I was always a morning person, this change for me was difficult. Bob Marley wrote a song that a hungry man is an angry man, and my song would be that a sleepy woman is a mad woman.

FRIDAY THE THIRTEENTH ON A THURSDAY THIS YEAR

For those who are superstitious, Friday the thirteenth may mean something different as to how they conduct themselves and their business for that day. To me it had no special meaning. For me it could be any day that I have interpreted as a bad day, regardless of the date. This day, I wanted to argue; I wanted to snap.

I'm cranky if I haven't slept well. My body hurts too, and I read different reasons between the lines as the causes for my aches and pains. At times I turned in bed for so long and could not find a comfortable position to sleep. I would have back pain, hip pain, shoulder pain, and/or neck pain. I would change from bedroom to living room and back to bedroom.

The only positive side of not getting enough sleep on one night was that I would be so tired the next day, so I would end up sleeping well the following night.

URINE, YOU'RE IN

One bad thing about having an accent is that people misunderstand what you are saying sometimes.

I can say, "urine," and someone may think that I have said, "You are in."

If you had to use a toilet after me, and still a little bit of my leftover urine smell remained, you would have guessed you were on a farm and not in my toilet.

"What kind of animal was in here?" you would ask.

I have asked myself too, during the first and the second trimester. No matter what amount of water I drink, that smell cannot be washed out, and it still has some kind of a funky odor.

It was also a different smell on different days. It was not consistently stinky, so that, if you went to a toilet after me, you could definitely say, "Aha, someone is pregnant."

THE SIZE DOES MATTER.
"SMALLER IS BETTER," SHE SAID.

It sometimes takes me a while to get some things I've read or seen, and, maybe two days later, the lightbulb goes on off in my brain. Then things make sense, and I can say, "Aha, I get it now."

This time it took me an entire month to say, "Aha, I get it." It was when I had the 3-D ultrasound. The only thing I remember was that Baby is cute and that he looks like his father. Finally that lightbulb started to glow in my brain, and I made some useful sense out of that visual image. If the boy looks like his father, then he will have other features like his father. For example, he will have his father's build.

Of course I am guessing these things. What Mother Nature will create, and how the genes will play their role, I don't know. At least it is comforting for me to think right now that the baby will not be taking after some uncle who was a giant with extralarge shoulders and a big head.

I am a little bit taller than my boyfriend. Who would think that I would appreciate this feature now during my pregnancy? I guess anything can be appreciated just to get peace of mind and to relax a bit. I have to find positive things in order to worry less about the labor.

Does a smaller baby mean easier labor and less pain?

Some women describe the pain of labor as like cramps during a menstrual period.

I don't think so. It can't be that good. I can live with that pain, not that it is pleasant, but it is endurable. If that is the intensity of the pain, then why do they make a big deal about it?

There has to be more to it; otherwise, I would not be scared of it.

Is it that I am scared of the unknown?

Or is it the thought that the pain may last for twenty-four hours?

Or is it the complications than can occur during the birth that could endanger me or the baby?

Yes, yes, yes, is the answer to all.

THE SIZE DOES MATTER
"BIGGER IS BETTER," HE SAID.

The shape of my body is, of course, different, so I don't think of myself as sexy or in good shape or anything like I could have described myself before the pregnancy. I just think of myself now as pregnant. There is the body, and there is the stomach, and that´s all there is to it.

My boyfriend, on the other hand, finds me even more attractive now.

He likes the size of my boobs, a little extra weight on my behind, and my wider hips. He even suggested that I should remain so after giving birth. The way he hugs now is by grabbing and touching everything as quickly as he can, before I start complaining that something hurts or that I am not comfortable and how he should stop that nonsense.

He almost got carried away a few times with the sucking of my breasts. My left boob suffered and paid the price, because she is bigger, and he likes her more. I tried to tolerate the pain and was successful at it for a while, because my tits were not so sensitive in the second trimester, thus I could actually enjoy his games a bit. But he kept on sucking and sucking, until I said something in order to stop him.

What really matters is that he wasn´t mad at me, and I wasn´t mad at him.

CRYING BABY

Does it ever happen that a mother accidently rolls over on her infant sleeping right next to her?

I doubt that. There has to be something subconsciously embedded in her mind that her baby is there; it has to be automatic. When the baby sleeps in another room, Mom can hear the baby cry and wake up instantly. Some mothers can get up even a few seconds before the baby starts to cry, because mother's intuition tells her that there is something wrong.

Fathers, on the other hand, can sleep through the cry of their own baby. I wonder why that is?

Was it maybe the fact that, during the hunting days, men spent less time with the children than the mothers, so the frequencies men hear at night are different than that of a woman's ear? I wonder what other couples would say to this question and if they would blame each other, arguing over of who is a better parent and who is the one to get up in the middle of the night to feed the baby.

TOTAL FOOD CONSUMPTION

On your mark, ... ready, set, and eat.

So what did I end up eating and consuming in the first six months of my pregnancy? This is not a wild guess but an actual estimation:

About 170 bananas, over 160 apples, 150 kiwis, 140 bread rolls, 130 eggs, 120 tomatoes, 110 pickles, 70 peppers, 60 carrots, 50 avocados, 40 cucumbers, 30 mangos, 20 papayas, 10 pineapples, 20 watermelons, 30 honeydew melons, 40 pears, 50 peaches, 200 strawberries, 200 cherries, 150 raspberries, 30 celery sticks, 40 raw red beets, 30 zucchinis, 10 pumpkins and squashes, 5 kg (about 11 pounds) of chestnuts, 30 kg (66 pounds) of potatoes, 10 kg (22 pounds) of onions, 2 kg (4.4 pounds) of garlic, 20 grapefruits and oranges, 30 pomegranates, 20 kg (about 44 pounds) of fish, 2 kg (4.4 pounds) of parsley, 10 kg (about 22 pounds) of cabbage, 10 kg (22 pounds) of broccoli, 5 kg (11 pounds) of sauerkraut, 20 kg (44 pounds) of green salad, 10 kg (22 pounds) of walnuts, 10 kg (22 pounds) of almonds, 100 liters (about 106 quarts or 26.5 gallons) of tea, 100 gallons of water, 2 buckets (4 pounds) of ice cream, 15 kg (33 pounds) of oatmeal, 5 kg (11 pounds) of corn meal.

LUCKY ME!

My life is pretty hectic, and this was my first quiet weekend spent at home since I got pregnant. Wow. Six months later and finally I could stay at home for two days and not think about if this weekend we were driving to my boyfriend's place or if we were going to a birthday party at a friend's house or if we were shopping for apartment accessories, baby clothes, or if, or if …

We could not stay put for one single weekend before this one. It was always one thing after another. And it always involved planning what to bring and pack up from the fridge. So many times, things have made a round trip from one fridge to another, and maybe next weekend again, back and forth.

Before the end of Sunday afternoon, I could almost say that I was bored. I even read something in German, to improve my knowledge of the language. Vacuumed a bit. Woo-hoo. Prepared lunch for Monday. Ooh la la. Boring stuff, right? But very important to notice because it meant that I was relaxed and had energy to do those things.

The most important thing was to eat healthy, drink tea, meditate, and do tai chi twice in a day. Is that too much to ask? Well, yes, it is, because it is simple. And simple things are always hard to figure out. The worse feeling is when I have no energy and know that doing tai chi would give me more energy, but I just can't do it. Same as with eating. I could be hungry but have no energy to prepare the food, which would in return give me the energy.

While bored and relaxed, I figured out one more thing! Remember how I already said that sometimes it takes me a few days or weeks to realize something? I think in school they call it a higher order of thinking skills. I have the knowledge, and I can understand it, but today I was able to analyze, evaluate, and see the big picture of how lucky I am to be in my shoes. Like someone used to say,

"It is good to be me." Or, when asked how you are today, the answer is, "Better than I deserve."

I will be working for only one more month. After that, I take saved-up vacation time for the rest of the year, with end-of-the-year holidays. In the New Year, I take a vacation again for one more week, because the calendar year changes, so now I get new days to take off. Then my family leave kicks in.

So here is the lucky-me part. I have days all to myself and the baby, before the birth, and I am talking about days and days and days: twenty + thirty-one + sixteen. That is sixty-six days, or little over two months to prepare myself mentally and physically for the baby's arrival.

I have heard a lot about the third trimester, and I am sure there will be many days when I will feel miserable and be cranky and have days of no sleep, and, and, and ...

At least I would have ways to manage it better. Why? Because we are taking work out of the equation. Another good part is that I will have the same pay during that time, plus two months after the birth of full pay or close to it. So no money worries, no work worries. The winter will be at its peak time too, so I would not be dressing and undressing for half an hour each day, riding a bicycle in freezing weather or waiting for a bus during cold, rainy or windy days.

I will not need to rush in the morning with my meditation and do a sloppy job in the evening. I could even add in a few sessions of acupuncture into my nonbusy schedule at the end of my pregnancy. All of that will make me more prepared for the birth than a normal working woman gets a chance to do in any other country, like in the USA.

Maybe I will say out loud one day that I love Germany, and that I love my job because of all benefits that I get from both. Even if I was a complete mess and out of shape, after two months there would still be hope for me to have a better chance of a normal and fast delivery. Maybe this is all my wishful thinking, but positive thinking can also get me somewhere.

It is kind of sad that the facts were there, and I had all this information in my head, but the pressure and stress were there too, and I couldn't think straight. So it took one long, boring weekend at home to have nothing else to do but figure it all out and finally say, "Relax. Everything will be all right."

LOVE HAS NO BORDERS, ONLY DIFFERENT HATS

My Tai Chi Master would wear many hats while I was learning techniques from him. Sometimes he also wore a hat as a best friend, as a father, and other times he would give me no breaks and would not listen to my moanings. That is when he would wear his hard-ass hat. Regardless of what hat he wore or I wore for the day, we always shared a mutual respect, with a lot of universal love.

After I told him that I was pregnant, he instantly started wearing his father hat. I could tell he was now a little worried about me, because he started calling me more frequently. If I was acting edgy in the previous phone call, he would point that out in the next one and ask if I was doing better than the last time.

I did not want him to worry about me, but I would have loved to have him nearby me, not as a father figure as much as a Tai Chi Master. Although he was not present with me physically in the past few months, his spirit was with me every time I would practice tai chi. Somehow everything started to come back. All the little details he would point out to me were now my focus during my stretches and exercises.

It is funny what pain can do. Pain can make you remember things that you thought you had forgotten or didn't even know that you had known them. The pain in my hips made me remember a lot of things he used to teach me. Who would think that I would appreciate his teachings ten years later more than I appreciated them back then? Who would have thought that I would push myself harder to do stretches for longer periods of time, and enjoy them, instead of being pushed by him and complaining about it?

The most adorable thing I have heard during my pregnancy was from him, when he said he was planning on writing a letter to my son. My Tai Chi Master wanted to write about the world my son was being brought into. I can´t wait to read that letter.

MORE SLEEP DOES NOT EQUAL MORE REST

I am losing the experience of what it means to be rested. It used to mean a good night of sleep, with a minimum of eight hours of uninterrupted sleep. If I am lucky, maybe in an eleven-hour period spent in bed, I get, on average, eight hours of sleep in between the toilet breaks every two hours. In the first trimester, I used to look at the clock to see what time it was. Now I can tell by the amount of liquid in my bladder, when I go to empty it, how many hours ago was the last time I got up for the toilet.

The other thing which didn't make sense is how soon after I get up in the morning that I would feel tired. I used to feel tired after at least half a day of work or after a good meal or some good exercise. Now it can mean after a few minutes of arriving at the office.

A few times it happened because my blood pressure was low, so, of course, that could also cause tiredness. The quickest and, to me, the tastiest way to increase my blood pressure is by adding more salt to my food. And, boy, how much do I like the taste of salty food. It is also well-known that salt retains water in the body. I have noticed after my few oversalted dinners that I would go to the toilet less at night, but it did not help the added thirst, so I still ended up drinking water in the middle of the night.

After so many months of pregnancy, and after so many attempts and experiments to increase my energy level, there were just days that I couldn't do anything about it.

Sleeping became more difficult because my body parts hurt while lying down, and I could not find a comfortable position to sleep. My hips were hurting if lying on my side, my butt cheeks if I was on my back, and the muscles of my upper legs if in a bent position. Sometimes my ankles felt swollen and achy, and most of the time my stomach was hurting. I had multiple flavors of pain: bladder, uterus, ovaries. Sometimes my underpants felt too tight, so I would remove them in the middle of the night.

I have changed pillows, my sleeping wardrobe, switched from bed to sofa. Sleeping with the window open or sleeping with the window closed also made no difference in the way I felt in the morning. *Tired* was the answer, no matter what.

I knew there was a positive side to that, which was all a beautiful plan by Mother Nature. If we were able to produce the babies any quicker, then we would not be used to this up-and-down business. Guess who we would like to blame in the middle of the night for not being sound asleep? We would blame the babies. I know it sounds sick, and I know that's who my neighbors will blame in the middle of the night, when they hear the sound of a crying baby.

I, on the other hand, will be the only one well trained to be up and will be glad that I am up. At least I will have someone to look at, someone to feed, someone to sing to, and someone to kiss. It beats the time now spent in bed, unable to sleep because I am worried about the baby and worried about how many more hours I have before getting up and going to work in the morning.

LAST PAIR OF PANTS, YIKES!

From any angle that I look at my body, my build looks normal. From the back, I look as if I have no extra weight, and I don't even look pregnant. From the front my legs still look very sporty and in shape. It is only my stomach that grew and my hips that extended proportionally with the boobs.

However, the baby already weighs over two pounds, and he has been doubling in size every month for the past three months. So when we add the ingredients inside the stomach that keep him alive, then one could guess that I am not that small either.

Yesterday I wore pants that had been somewhat comfortable for the past two months. I wore them last week, and they felt a bit tight. I wore them this week again, and sitting in the office all day actually caused some pain, because those pants felt tighter than the previous week. I have three more pairs left that are one size bigger than those pants!

I would not be making such a big deal of this if I was not at the last size for the slim-mama department. It does not bother me that I will need to switch now to the XL section or the XXL section, if the selection or the fit was good. The problem is that everything I have looked at so far is really designed for the women who are large everywhere. Not only from the front, but I mean from *everywhere*.

The clothes that I have tried on really do not fit me. This is not the time to complain about my looks, I know. This is the time to hope that I don't explode in size all over and only continue growing in my belly. That´s the story for my pants, but what annoys me is that even my tops, the stretchy clothes, started to be so tight.

Once I am on vacation, I will not be wearing any dress pants or work pants for a while. I will make sure that all of my outfits are loose, and preferably half of my days will be spent in pajamas or a bathrobe. Only my exercise clothes will be worn once per day to go for a nice walk, but I will not be sitting in anything tight, pushing against my stomach or squeezing my thighs and making me achy every day after work.

ANOTHER CONFESSION AND A WHITE LIE

I said that I would stop reading about things that make me worry more. I still ended up reading some interesting facts, and, yes, they got me worried now too.

During my first trimester I was freaking out about the idea of not being able to breast-feed, being forced to use baby formula, so I was researching the alternatives to cow's milk and/or soy baby formula. In the second trimester I was researching making labor easier and quicker, and the more knowledge I accumulated, the more worried I became. When I stopped researching, all of a sudden I stumbled on the relevant information that made me even more worried about the labor pain.

Breast-feeding sounds painful too, and I am not referring to sore nipples.

It is not that I am scared of not having enough milk. What I have read is that breast-feeding takes so much energy out of mother, because her biosystem makes so much effort to give life to that baby that she may even lose 4 percent of her brain weight or volume. I forgot which one.

Now what the hell am I reading? If this is really true, then I am screwed.

Do I have enough brain that I can even afford to lose some now?

Or is this the case of no brain, no pain.

I don't know, but, to me, this picture is starting to look wrong. Really. Think about it.

Women are usually not worried about losing weight, and it is something they look forward to.

But losing brain weight?

Oh, my gosh.

Number one, I already have enough issues with my energy from pregnancy, and I was looking forward to having that child next to me after the birth and getting my energy back just from joy. Wrong. Think again if you are breast-feeding.

Do I have to repeat myself for the thousandth time and ask again?

Where are all these women with pregnancy knowledge when I need them?

How come no one else made a big deal out of this and did something about it?

Am I just going to keep quiet?

Or just write my mom back home about it and leave it at that?

No, no, no. You are all wrong, sisters, moms, women, aunts, ladies.

Number two, how can I afford to lose more of my brain cells? I have lost enough. Look what I have turned into. If I haven't convinced you by now, then I don't know what I will do. Do I need to write a book afterward, so you can be your own judge and compare notes?

You know, when our parents used to say how much they sacrificed for their children, they never said anything about sacrificing brain cells, for gosh sakes. C´mon, kiddo. I have heard of cases when parents donate a kidney to their child, but the brain? Who will raise my child then, if I have less brain cells?

THIRD TRIMESTER

LANDING

MONTH 7 - DECEMBER

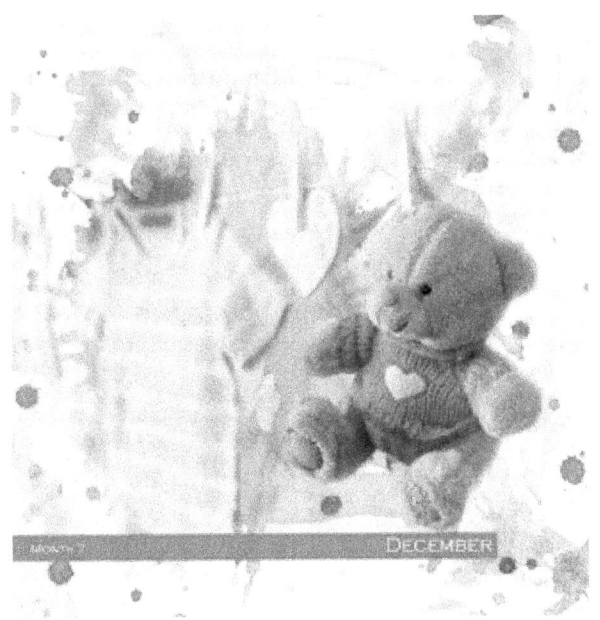

WARNING! YOU NEED TO SLOW DOWN.

A few days ago my boyfriend caught me vacuuming the house at full speed. He looked around and added up other things I had accomplished over the past few hours, and he was not happy to see me move around as if I were not pregnant.

Today we are at the full seventh-month mark. The good news is, it took me only a few days to digest his suggestion and to finally admit that this is not a time to joke around. Premature babies like to come in the seventh month.

The first part of the plan to slow down was to have only one thing to do for the day and nothing else. For example, I will only be washing clothes that day, and not cleaning the bathroom, mopping the floors, or organizing the closet. While we are here, let´s rearrange the kitchen too, and we women are well capable of doing that spontaneously.

The second thing on the plan was also to use this seven-month mark as the time for my body to prepare for labor. I have been delaying long enough not thinking about it too much, not being fully informed, not being prepared for Dah Day!

Coincidently last night I also observed how my tai chi moves are totally out of control. My steps are too big, and I don't take a half step when required. I am still doing the same stances and moving my body, as I am in full-form, fully stretched all the time, and as flexible as one can be.

In reality, my balance is off, and my moves are more mechanical than intuitive. I used to listen to my body only and go with the flow. With the baby now, my center of gravity is at a different place, so I should not be using my old center of gravity to balance. Now I have to listen to the baby.

Why is it so hard to slow down? Is that another pregnancy side effect?

NEW TASTE

Winter is approaching, and the grocery stores have fewer selections of fruits and vegetables. My baby has already tasted everything offered on the shelves, and my routine diet must be somewhat boring for him at this stage. My cravings for overly spicy food are now behind me, although I still like foods hot. Now the baby responds only to sour things that I eat, and I can feel him kick and move right away.

Lemongrass tea did it this morning too, and I was happy to find something that excites my boy. He'd never tasted lemongrass, so I felt his kicks after I drank tea early in the morning. Usually he is not even up at those hours, but I could tell he wanted a new taste.

I got his kick out of it, so I'm happy.

GIFTS FROM MR. MAILMAN

A few days ago four things were delivered for the baby from Mr. Mailman. Thanks to online shopping and weekly advertisements in the mail, I have scored a good deal on a baby crib and stroller. Two other pieces came with the stroller: a Moses basket and a car seat for the baby.

I haven't even unpacked the trio stroller set package yet, because I am sure there is some assembly required, so am I staying out of my minitoolbox. Right now I am also thinking that the trio set can be put together as one unit, so that the basket is part of the stroller in the same way the car seat is part of the stroller.

An update! (Two hours later ...)

Everything is sweet, and I didn't even need any kind of a tool to put the pieces together. Almost everything came assembled, so there was not much to put together. I have left the small technical details for my boyfriend to finish, like installing the wheels properly and ensuring everything is tight and secure.

I am a satisfied customer. The car seat can also be part of the stroller, so they have really engineered this well. And where have I been? Probably this technology is twenty years old. Well, obviously, I have not been in the baby business for that long.

GIFTS FROM MAMA

I want to knit a little baby hat, because it will be cold when we are making our trip from the hospital to home. Since the wool may be too harsh for his skin, I will probably line the inside of the hat with cotton, which also means that this hat will be extra warm, a very useful thing to have at that time.

While I am knitting, I should also make a small pair of gloves and socks. OK, you can laugh now, thinking that all the baby outfits will be sewed by me, and there will be nothing commercial in the baby's closet. Take it easy. I don't even own a sewing machine and don't know how to sew. Of course I will be buying outfits. I know my friends will be bringing presents for him, so we will end up with a collection of things from the store anyway.

I just laughed out loud. I am picturing my little boy looking like a little guy from a village with some kind of a funky woolen hat. Well, since my baby won't be getting any Armani newborn hats, gloves, and scarfs, then I will have to design my own. The good part about making these things is that I can later frame them as a shadow-box picture on the wall with a nice memory of my baby's coming-home outfit.

If I was expecting a first-time guest to spend the weekend or a few weeks with me, I would have prepared for them, ensuring the house was extra clean, stocking up on some favorite foods, posting a Welcome sign on the door maybe, doing something special to make this guest feel really at home.

My baby is not a guest, and he will be arriving home for the first time, so my extra little present is only to say, "Welcome home, baby."

MORE THAN A BOYFRIEND

Last year my boyfriend had a number of doctor's visits and medical tests. I admired his health concerns and that he took good care of himself by choosing to consult with different doctors. Today he called to let me know he would not be going to work tomorrow and then spending the night at my place, because he had a doctor's appointment.

I was worried more today about him than I was about his previous visits to the doctor. This made me realize that I feel different toward him than I did before I became pregnant.

Some time ago, years and years back, my smarty-pants self used to say:

"If I wanted to have a baby, I did not need a man around."

Now I am feeling different about that statement of mine.

Maybe it is half true. Maybe I don't need the man.

The baby does.

If it was someone else telling me this a year ago, I would probably be like:

"Ha? What? I don't get it."

If someone mistakenly said that a woman needs a *husband* instead of a *man*, I would have a whole heap of arguments about why people should never be married in the first place.

And look at me now.

How much my baby and my man have changed me.

We haven't even started playing the role of parents yet, but I like it already.

SLEEPLESS NIGHT

Today at work was the worst that I have felt when it comes to my energy level. Just last night I realized how little stress I get from my boyfriend. Last night he was not there, because he needs to see his family doctor first thing in the morning. I had a pretty much sleepless night, because I was worried about him.

I was not able to sleep for more than a few minutes before my bladder woke me, and I had to get up and empty it. Every time I woke up, I also cried for a while, because something nice would cross my mind about my boyfriend.

In the middle of the night, I felt like jumping on the train and going to his house. There was no train connection at that hour from my place. Then I thought about staying awake until morning and jumping on the first train. The next thing I knew, the alarm was waking me. My hormones were really out of whack. Should I just head to work or do I go to the train station?

To call work and say I was not coming in, and then to see my own doctor to ask for a sick day was too much for me, so I headed to work. I packed a small suitcase, in case my boyfriend calls me and needs to spend the night at the hospital, so I am ready to leave work at any time and head his way.

Once I was at work, it bothered me to sit there and just wait for his phone call. The worst part is that my office looked like a conference room as I walked in, and I was hoping to be alone. My office mate explained that four more people were here for a conference call. I said that this was an office and not a conference room. I am sure my look said more than that. I was tired, had on no makeup, and was obviously pregnant.

Just around the corner were two large meeting rooms, fully available for the whole day, and, by the time I came back to give my office mate that update, half of the participants had already found their way out, and the other half was getting ready to leave. After my bathroom trip, two minutes later, my office was empty.

My dilemma came to an end, when my boyfriend phoned. I ended up jumping on the train as soon as he said that he had more doctor visits scheduled for the next few days.

I was glad that he did not end up in the hospital. To be there with him, and for him, I knew it would do more than good for both of us, instead of me wondering, at my own house, how he was doing.

Before he even finished his first doctor's appointment for the day, I had already found my way to the waiting room to meet him. His smile told me everything and how glad he was to see me. I think at that moment he forgot he was sick, and the only thing that mattered was that I was next to him.

MAMA ON HORMONES

How did Mother Nature envision the role of hormones, and what kind of a tune is she playing? Both are still a mystery to me. For six months I have been experiencing their dance and still don't know the name of the song.

Why was I so off balance, jumpy, sensitive, and vicious in a programmed hormones' play by Mother Nature? Was it really to protect the newborn or was my behavior just part of my horrible character?

For my boyfriend to put up with all my nasty business must have been really hard. In the end I think I have become a better person.

MONTH 8 - JANUARY

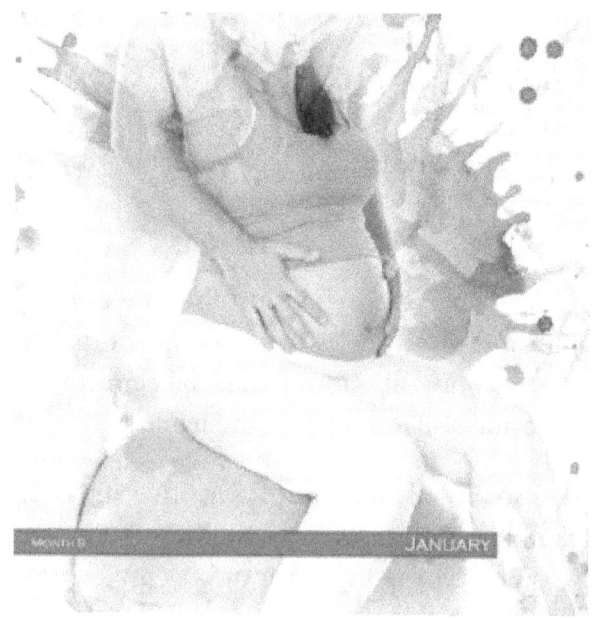

THERE ARE NO BAD HORMONES, ONLY MY MOOD AND CHARACTER.

So many times in my pregnancy I have blamed and referenced hormones as a potent drug and the cause of all evil. It is now time to admit my own faults and confess that I can be a wicked beast that only my mother can love. There are times when my mother can't love that monster either, but there is one person who can still forgive, forget, and love me, as if nothing has happened. My lovely boyfriend.

On this one particular occasion my misbehavior was triggered by waiting an extra five minutes in the cold weather after work. I was wrong to asking him to pick me up in the first place, when I could have walked my lazy ass to the bus stop.

So he had to pick up the drama queen.

He had to listen to my bitching during the entire drive, which was luckily short, so it didn't last more than ten minutes. In this case only ten minutes was probably relatively long for him, because he was hearing me go on and on ...

"I don´t like waiting at the bus stop in this weather. It is better to ride my bicycle. It is also safer to ride my bike, because, if it is freezing and I am walking, then I could fall down and injure myself, while the bike lanes are cleaner and safer to ride on."

This talk was probably to give him a hard time for asking me not to ride my bicycle anymore, since it was dangerous, and I could injure myself and the baby.

My mood changed quickly, and my head started to cool off. The guilt trip then kicked in. My emotions rocked from nasty woman to a sensitive human being. Now I was crying.

Why was I crying?

I was crying for realizing that my hormones were not the cause of my behavior. My bad ass thinks it is always right, and it has priority over everything and everybody.

Wasn´t I the same person just a few days ago crying because I felt sorry for him that he was sick?

What is wrong with me, and how could I forget that this man will be there for me and the baby more than anyone else? Why was I acting like he was nobody to me and that I can just say whatever I want, whenever I want?

I swear, any other person would either talk back to me or at least make me realize that I am wrong. Better yet, any other man would just stop the car and tell me to get the hell out—pregnant or not, it wouldn't matter. Any other man would just leave my ass forever.

Have I really accomplished anything with my anger, temper, and mean character? Even when I was nasty toward nasty people, who probably deserved to see me in that state, it never helped solve anything. Now how can I think it would work with the nicest man in the whole world?

My hormones were there first, before my temper arrived, and I need to give a little more respect to their role and function.

So next time I find an excuse to blame my hormones, I better check myself and my own actions first.

WHAT ABOUT FUTURE FATHER?

My boyfriend's tolerance for my occasional harshness was humongous even before the pregnancy. For some reason I couldn't do anything obnoxious to him that would make him turn his head and say good-bye forever. He always found a place in his heart to forgive me and to forget.

I wondered so many times, how can he love me so much? Is it because I make delicious dinners for him?

He should not take all that crap from me.

He should not be hurt so much, so many times. I deserve to be given more hell.

During my pregnancy we grew closer. I started having more empathy. My complaints changed. I used to sound like a broken record in the morning and say things like:

"I am tired and couldn't sleep, because I had to get up one hundred times to potty."

Later on I would ask him if he slept well and if I woke him

up while getting up. Before it never crossed my mind that he could also be tired from a lack of sleep, because I had to get up to use the toilet and disturbed him.

What about those days when I woke myself up with my loud snoring? How did he react to my snoring? On many occasions he would touch me to see if that would make my snoring stop or at least make it quieter. He never tried to wake me up and say, "Turn on the other side. You are snoring too much, and I can't sleep."

What a wonderful man to have beside me. What if he was like me?

WHERE AM I MORE COMFORTABLE AT NIGHT?

At times I couldn't sleep because my boyfriend was snoring, so I would run to the living room and sleep on the couch. If he woke up before I had to use the toilet, he would look for me in the living room and would wake me up, asking if I was doing OK.

Then I would feel guilty for leaving him alone in bed, so I would join him again in the bedroom. Usually he would fall back asleep within minutes, and I would be turning over and over again for the next half hour. By that time I would need to get up and use the toilet again. So I would run back to the living room and try to sleep on the couch once more. Sleep was more important than comfort.

By the end of the second trimester, the bond with my

boyfriend was getting stronger, and his snoring did not bother me. I would rather not sleep than be alone on the couch.

MULTIPLE CHOICES OF PREGNANCY'S SIDE EFFECTS

Side effects perform stuffs that are not expected or envisioned. In medical terms it is usually referred to as an unwanted effect of a drug. If you have read the first chapter of this book, then you know the drug that I am referring to in this case is hormones.

Before I summarize my pregnancy's side effects, first let´s change the technical term of *frequent urination* to *constant urination*. Why not? It makes no difference to you, does it?

Now for the summary of my side effects while pregnant:

Frequent visits to the gynecologist was one of those side effects that I got used to during the nine months. I have had more visits to Lady Doctor this year than I have had in my lifetime.

Feeling cranky and tired. Feeling supertired and exhausted. Insomnia. Going crazy, coming back, and going crazy again. Loss of breath. Loss of appetite. Constipation. Gas. Smelly urine. Dizziness. No hair growth for months. Too much appetite and weight gain. Swollen breasts. Painful breasts caused by squeezing them into too-small bra. Tight pants and shopping for extralarge clothes. Bladder infection. Yeast infection. Snoring. Nightmares. Bleeding gums. Back pain. Headaches. Increased vaginal discharge. Bloody nose. Drooling while sleeping.

Let me thank Mother Nature for giving me only, and I repeat, only these side effects.

Why do I say *only*?

Well, because I have survived, and it could have been worse.

There is a much longer list of all other side effects that I could have had, and luckily I did not. Morning sickness, for example. I have read about the others, and some of them I have never heard of before. So let me say that I feel lucky for having my set. This is not to say that it was easy.

Would I do it all over again?

CURIOUS PUPPY FINDING THE EXIT DOOR

My baby makes me laugh so much already, so I know he will be a funny character and have a good sense of humor when he grows up.

He is so curious now. He is very busy pulling on the umbilical cord and doing who-knows-what with it.

A coworker told me a story when his wife was pregnant, about how she ended up making an emergency visit to the doctor because she stopped feeling the baby's movements for hours. This was now close to her due date, and Mama couldn't feel or hear the baby's heartbeat. The doctor was happy to announce that her daughter was doing fine and was just sleeping.

Last night my baby boy found the exit door or the magic passage that he will use to come out on this side of our world. I literally felt his little hand touching the membrane. At first it was ticklish to me, and he made me laugh, but a few seconds later I was concerned that he would punch the door and come out prematurely.

I like to think that he will keep these qualities and end up as a smart and curious little puppy.

MORE SIMILAR DREAMS

I have a reoccurring dream. It starts a few minutes after the baby's birth. The doctor hands me the baby, and I start breast-feeding right away. My nipples feel the pressure from Baby's strong sucking. The baby eats for a while, but I want to pick him up for a burp. His face is covered in milk, including his neck.

Now the weird part of the dream starts. The doctor was satisfied with his tests, so now the baby is supposed to go back in my womb. I am, of course, against that idea, because the baby looks good; he is healthy; I have milk for him, and there is no reason for him to go back. The doctor is in a dilemma also, because he forgot how much water he took from my stomach and how much he is supposed to put back. Finally he decides not to return the baby where he came from. What a relief that was for me.

BABY DOES IT.

This baby loves to ride in any kind of vehicle. He usually gets active during the first few minutes of car movement. I think he likes the combination of motion with the music. Usually when the car stops at the traffic light, he will kick, as if asking, "Why did we stop moving?"

As the baby is getting stronger every day, I can also feel the difference in his moves and kicks. At first he would only kick a few times, but now I can feel him move from one side to another. When he turns, it is hard not to notice where his shoulder may be, his head, or his butt, because I feel different parts of his body traveling inside me.

This morning we have had the longest playtime so far, and it must have lasted for more than twenty minutes. I was lying on my back in bed, and I was gently rubbing and making circles with my fingers on one side of my belly. He responded. Then I moved my fingers toward the middle of my stomach, and he responded again in the same spot as my fingers. I repeated the moves at different locations, and he responded accordingly.

Then I decided to stop and see if he was interested in playing more games. He was moving around again to the point that he made me laugh, because I felt his feet, as if he was running and getting ready to make a big flip and tumble a full 360 degrees.

I don't even know why I laugh, and it is not because it tickles me. It is just the sudden surprise of feeling his strength and feeling my connection with him. Now I can see why parents are proud of anything their children do. I am now proud of my little one because he plays with me, or at least that is my own interpretation of this game. Of course all of this could be my imagination, but, as far as I can see, the pattern is there, and we are communicating with each other.

AN ERR GEE (ENERGY). TIRED OF BEING TIRED.

We are in the third trimester and close to my due date. My stomach is not only getting bigger but also feeling bigger. I can tell that my days of high energy are over, and the last trimester is starting to take a toll on me. I am feeling what my friends warned me about. The lack of energy in the morning is the same as I had in the first trimester.

GENERAL DISCRIMINATION

The way my pregnancy has been going, I feel lucky. My only complaints were about the side effects, but I feel good about having the child and what the future will bring us.

I can think of comparing this pregnancy to my childhood. If someone asked me what kind of childhood I had, and, in case I had no time to talk for hours, I would have said that I had a happy childhood. If I had more than a few hours to explain, the story from a happy child would probably shift slowly to some not-so-happy memories.

It is the same with my pregnancy. I know that I will later think of my pregnancy as happy times, because I have not had any kind of medical complications.

Will I also remain quiet and not do anything about improving the lives of pregnant women like most other fellow pregnant women have done in the past? Will I do something for future pregnant ladies, who will end up going through and dealing with the same difficulties as the rest of us pregnant women? Going to work, feeling guilty for calling in sick, and struggling to stay calm when we want to scream at the top of our lungs?

Why do we want to accept something that should not be acceptable?

Let me get back to a simple question.

Why are women not demanding more rights during pregnancy?

Why, in some countries, do pregnant women get more time off before and after childbirth, while in other countries the time spent with the baby is different?

Why do so many women keep quiet and pretend as if it was easy to grow a new organ (a placenta) inside their bodies that will help with the growth of a small human?

TALK SHOWS FOR PREGNANT WOMEN?

How come there is no radio talk show for pregnant women?

Or a TV show? Or a pregnant woman hosting a show?

Or a QVC–like channel only for pregnant women?

There are so many stupid shows with lame topics that we have all watched and wasted our time in front of the TV. The hosts will cover anything and everything. Most of the time in the States, they make fun of the politicians, entertainment celebrities, and other people who are in the spotlight at that time, for who-knows-what-reason. We have seen all kinds of crazy talk shows, some of them run by real freaks too.

Yet we pregnant women are not ready to talk about our experience freely and say what bothers us.

The celebrity women will pop up on TV for a few seconds and just announce that they are pregnant. Most of the time they are hiding, and not only physically hiding but also hiding the whole story of what is going on while they are pregnant. Some of them will be followed by paparazzi to snap a shot of their belly or make a big deal on the trends and wardrobe styles for maternity clothes. The paparazzi are interested in their weight gain, so they can later track them and show the before and after. Is that really interesting?

Hundreds of things experienced by millions of women during pregnancy remain hidden and buried with the rest of the old, mostly forgotten items usually stored in a basement or a dungeon. Why, I ask?

CHECKLIST BEFORE YOU TOUCH MY BABY

Here is a list of questions that a person will need to answer before touching my baby. Part of the list will be posted on the main entrance door to my home. Part of the list will be posted on the baby crib and the stroller. Maybe some questions (Q) will be totally personal. There is a reason (R) for all of that, so let me spell them out too.

(Q1) Do you have kids of your own?

(R) If the person hasn't carried a small baby, I will not let them practice on my newborn.

(Q2) Do you have a flu/cold? Any other known contagious diseases?

(R) Obviously you came here to cause harm by spreading your germs, so please turn around and go back to where you came from.

(Q3) When was the last time you brushed your teeth?

(R) My baby may not be strong enough and know how to turn his head quickly to the other side due to unpleasant odors.

(Q4) Do you smoke?

(R) Baby does not know how to say *paheeeww*.

(Q5) Have you ever done any harm to any kind of animal?

(R) So I can kick the person out of the house without even asking any further questions.

(Q6) Do you have a tendency to do things and forget that you have done them?

(R) The person may forget that they are holding a precious baby and daydream about who-knows-what.

(Q7) Is your cell phone off?

(R) Your full attention should be on holding the baby and not who may be calling.

(Q8) Have you had an alcoholic beverage today?

(R) I don't want your physical reflexes impaired while holding my baby, and I don't need my baby inhaling your drunken breath.

(Q9) Do you have anything bad to say about Baby's mother or father?

(R) If yes, step away from the baby, because you may try to avenge some unfinished business.

(Q10) Did any of the questions annoy you?

(R) If yes, then step away from the baby, because you are annoying us already.

ITCHING, SCRATCHING, AND PAIN IN THE …

Another side effect is that my skin is so dry that it could be used to soak up wet spills. Dry skin itches too, and it itches in weird places and at the wrong times. I could be in the middle of the meeting, and, all of a sudden, I feel like scratching my thighs or the muscles right above my boobs.

Now what´s up with my tailbone, and how come I started getting pain there recently too?

I know, sometime in my childhood, I hit that area when falling off a sled while sliding downhill. It was bruised and hurt for a couple weeks. I do not remember having pains there after that incident. Yes, I have been sitting for a prolonged time due to my office job, but I don't think I am developing some kind of arthritis now in my tailbone.

The only explainable reason—or, better yet, a wild guess—is that I have added too much weight to my frame, and working in the office from nine to five probably adds a little extra pressure on that area. That means now I am making conscious decisions on how to position my legs while sitting down. This also means that sleeping on my back is also painful, in case I put too much pressure on my tailbone.

Since I have been sleeping on my left-hand side, as many websites recommend doing during pregnancy, my left side feels sore. Everything hurts, sometimes even my left ear from the pillow, plus my stomach, my thighs, my knees. Last night I tried to sleep on my right-hand side, and that didn't go so well. Needless to say I look like crap on this Monday morning, with dark circles under my eyes.

Is that a good reason to go home and not suffer at my office desk today? Saying that I have tailbone pain would not be a good idea. To say that I can't sit in my office anymore would be true.

My time-off request may backfire, when my boss responds that I am a pain in his tailbone.

IMMIGRANTS AND PREGNANT WOMEN

When it comes to discrimination as to immigrants and as to pregnant women, the answer is everything and nothing.

1. People look and sometimes stare.

I am still not used to having people look at me as if there was something wrong with me. Some people check me out, and some stare for a long time, as if I look really different because I am from another place. When someone stares at my stomach, for some reason that makes me uncomfortable. It is not that I am uncomfortable on my own and have issues with the way I look because I am pregnant. But just having someone look at my belly, somehow it makes me feel little, and I don't know why. Of course I could always approach the person and ask:

"What the fuck are you looking at? Never seen a pregnant woman before?"

2. Difficult to understand.

Most of the immigrants think differently due to their cultural backgrounds, and sometimes they may be hard to understand. Women in general are hard to understand. Pregnant women are impossible to understand.

3. Can't go back.

Just like immigrants who can't go back to where they are originally from, pregnant women can't go back to their original state (nonpregnant).

4. Rich woman, poor woman.

There are moments when immigrants feel like the happiest and luckiest people, as if they are so rich just because they are now in another country. Then there are times when the reality kicks in and makes them feel so poor. Pregnant women also have days when they feel like the richest women in the world because of their baby, and then, when they look around their environment that they are bringing the baby into, they may feel poor. And not poor from the viewpoint of money, just poor because of an emptiness inside them, regardless of how much money they have.

5. Wonder how they ended up here.

Some women may ask themselves how they ended up pregnant, when they know damn well how it happened. They got lucky! Immigrants can also believe in luck or that it took a miracle for them to end up in that kingdom.

6. If I had only known …

Sometimes there are regrets, but there is no way of going back. Acceptance is the final stage of adopting a new environment.

MIRRORS AND SCALES, PLEASE LIE TO ME

Tomorrow I must visit the doctor for a checkup. One more after that in three weeks, and then I am back on biweekly checkups.

I must remember to ask the nurse not to tell me how much I weigh. If I step on the scale, I can't see it anyway with my stomach, and she can just write it down in my chart, without announcing it loud and clear. I am afraid the number has changed from the last reading, which means I have gained more than X amount, and I don't want to hear any of that. It's not like we pregnant women don't have enough changes going on, and now I have to worry about that too.

The last visible change I had seen was last night in the mirror, while shaving my well-hidden, under-the-stomach part, which looked like it had gained some weight too. It looked very different from the last time I had checked it out. The poor thing had aged so quickly, and I really don't know what happened. As if it was in some kind of war zone. Wonder how it will look later, after the little one passes through?

ENGINEERING THE HAT

So I finally finished the little hat, and the knitting is completed. It took me at least five or six different stabs at it. I would start, not like something about it, and then start over again. Sometimes it was the wrong size, or sometimes the pattern never quite seemed right.

Although it may look small, I know it is still big enough at least to bring the little one home from the hospital. The hat's diameter is more than 10 cm, and, if a woman needs to open up 10 cm before delivery, that means, to me anyway, that the baby's head cannot be more than 10 cm in diameter. Can it?

The color of the hat is black with fluffy little firework-looking adornments ending in a beige color. At the beginning of this conception, everything was black, and yet the light will be at the end, so that is the meaning of the beige color. The first pattern is called "rice" in knitting language. This is because he was the size of a rice grain when I learned that I was pregnant during the first ultrasound.

There are a total of three patterns, and each pattern represents one of the trimesters.

The first pattern is all rough-looking, representing the first trimester; the second one is a smooth pattern, and the third one is intertwined with rough and smooth.

I CAN'T HANDLE THE LIES

During my pregnancy something would tick me off more than anything. It was the lies, and anyone and everyone who told them. Not that I enjoyed listening to lies before, but now I hated them with passion. My face would turn red, as if I was the one telling the lies. If I took part in the conversation to convince those liars how wrong they were, my voice would also get shaky, and I would start losing my voice.

After the lairs were long gone out of my sight, they would not be out of my mind. I would reprocess their lies in my head and preoccupy myself with those unacceptable things. I was really allergic to them, and it was a big energy drain for me. Why now?

Why was I taking so many lies so personally?

ENOUGH IS ENOUGH

Enough of my writing. Enough of my bitching. Enough of my two cents. Time for action.

I remember a lotto commercial with a guy riding a bicycle one way on a scenic road. A few seconds later, the same bike is on top of a car rack, and the guy is driving a Porsche in the opposite direction (after picking up his lotto money). The slogan was: if you wanted to win, you had to play.

Similarly, during election time, to encourage voters to get out and vote, the slogan went something like this: they can't bitch, if they don't vote. I have forgotten the exact wording of that slogan.

Now it is my time to wrap up the months-long bitching and do something once and for all about the way pregnancy is perceived socially, politically, and from one culture to another.

I know. I know. That means getting off my ass and doing something for a change.

Now is a good time for a confession.

I planned on editing this book before the baby was born and readying for publishing as soon as the baby arrived. My next writing project was to be called something along the lines of *Two Cents from a Woman without a Country*. This memoir will be about my previous life, how I moved twenty times while living in five different states in the USA, then on a Caribbean island for nine years, and lastly my move to Germany.

My third book was planned to be written before the end of the year. My mind was on a cookbook for pregnant woman and new moms during the child's first twelve months.

If I remember correctly, the way this book starts is with a remarkable question of what the world would look like if women had a choice of not working while pregnant. Sitting around on my ass, for sure, still sounds good, if I had enough money, but I am sure that would have gotten me nowhere. Still, I have to give something back to the community and help future moms.

I did not want to be like the rest of them.

Why is it that all women forget the pain once they hold their newborn?

I am not there yet, so I better deliver something bigger than just an eight-pound baby. Something that will be better for all women. A revolution? Not literally, more of a social change.

LAST DAY AT WORK

I did it.

My last day of work while pregnant, and I have survived. I can't say it is because I am a survivor. No, that's not the reason …

The real reason is because I did not quit two days ago. Seriously. Of course I would not do such a thing, but I wanted to call in sick. Do I really care at this point how many times I have called in sick and that I have the guts to do it again right before my vacation?

No. I have no shame; we know that already.

Do you want to know why I didn't feel like coming to work? There is a good reason for that. Trust me. To make matters worse, I hadn't slept well the night before. Remember how my clothes were getting smaller and smaller? Yes, everything was tight, and that was giving me stomach pains in the evening. My winter jacket was also too tight around my stomach, and it was too cold to wear it open.

They may not sound like good reasons to you, but, for me, it was a good reason to stay home.

WHAT DO POLITICS HAVE TO DO WITH PREGNANCY?

I am back at my desk. I am cleaning up not only my physical space, as if I am never coming back to work again, but I am also cleaning up my electronic space by deleting anything and everything personal that was on my computer.

Maybe I really will get lucky, and my book sells well. That's still not enough in my opinion to make a big difference for pregnant women everywhere, so I think the solution is to get into politics.

Did I ever want to get into politics?

Hell no.

I don't think I was loud enough.

Hell no!

Now that's much better.

But I can't forget that I am getting older, and things that we didn't like when we were younger can all of a sudden start to interest us. I didn't like spinach before either, but now I eat it.

I didn't like history as a school subject. Why? Because they were only teaching the WWI and WWII history, and we had to memorize dates written in those books. It took me twenty years later to like history.

Same with politics. I have been avoiding politics for more than twenty years. Religion too. I ran from them as far as I can.

And now I want to get into politics?

Well, the way I see it, I don't have a choice. If I want to change the world around me, the world of pregnant women, yes, I can do that with book writing and getting a reality show with a bunch of pregnant women running around. Would that be enough? I ask myself. Of course not.

So now I am shifting my gears. From wishing to be a lazy mom—sitting around at home and doing nothing but raising children—now I have a challenge.

The only two requirements would be that my baby is with me everywhere I go, and I can breast-feed whenever necessary.

Do you think that would be possible?

Of course not.

So let me say good-bye to the politics quick, because I still don't like the idea of me involved in that.

MY SUITS AND FASHION EVOLUTION

I don´t know which century I would have been the most comfortable in when it comes to outfits and the most appropriate clothing to wear during pregnancy. Would I be wearing skirts, pants, or skants?

I am not comfortable at all in my clothes. Only while standing up, some clothes have a comfortable feel, but, when I sit down or lay down, everything starts to become too tight.

For example, while sitting in a car, I used to put my hand under the waistline of my pants to stretch out my clothes and make more free space. That works for a short drive, but it became painful as my stomach got bigger. If someone were watching, of course, it would have looked suspicious, as if I was doing some other business.

The second option was to pull down my pants, now somewhere in the middle of my thighs. There is only one issue with that solution. Yes, the stomach is now free, but after a while, it becomes too tight for my thighs. I don't even care at this point if another vehicle would pull up next to ours and if someone would see me with my pants half down. It wouldn't be the first time either.

The same solution applies while at home, watching TV on the couch or trying to catch an afternoon nap. The pants and panties must come down halfway to my knees. I would cover up with the blanket so I didn't feel cold while half naked. Better yet, so I don´t get embarrassed in case a guest shows up at the house with my boyfriend, and all of a sudden I have to get up, half asleep, or forgot what I was wearing or not wearing.

Who would have thought that I could exceed the limits of stretchy clothing and that they can become tight too?

PEE PEE ODOR IS BACK AND THE H WORD

In the eighth month one of my very undesirable side effects was back. The urine odor. The toilet refreshers sitting inside the flushing tank and toilet bowl are not enough to cancel out that stink. OK, fine, but let´s address the real concern here. The hormones.

Yes, the hormones are the cause of the stinking pee. So what´s there to worry about?

Everything.

The body changes cause my pains and my killer mood.

I don't know how much more of the body changes I can take. I now have, as a result of hormones, the black nipples, one long dark line running in the middle of my stomach, stretching from my vagina almost all the way to my diaphragm, which I still don't know what it means. Another one showed up in a horizontal direction right under my boobs.

I still have frequent itching caused by my dry skin, an increase in vaginal discharge, bleeding gums, and pain in my joints due to the pregnancy weight gain.

On top of that, I also have a sharp pain in my breasts. I have tailbone pain from sitting, and I have pains in my belly from the extra pressure on my uterus, sometimes caused by the baby and sometimes caused by my daily activities. I have pain in my middle back, in my lower back, and sometimes I feel as if my hair hurts too.

My sleeping pattern is still disrupted because of the frequent urination. Luckily the mood changes are not as hyped up as in the first trimester, or at least that is the way it appears to me. My tiredness and exhaustion periods are also more bearable now, because I am not spending most of my day behind a desk at work, and I have more freedom on when to start my day and how to end it.

My concern is that my hormones will start acting up later, which means my behavior will be unbearable.

THE P, AS IN POSITIVE

There are still plenty of days and weeks left in those two final months of my pregnancy, but I have plenty to be grateful for. The baby is doing fine, and that´s really something to celebrate. His weight increased by 400 g (0.8 pounds) in the last two weeks, which is the same amount as my own weight increased. So I feel better that my weight is somewhat stable now, and I am not gaining five pounds or so every month, and my cravings have eased off a bit, almost to the point where I have no appetite. Of course I still get my energy drain, so planning my meals is helpful before the little prince takes the energy away from Mama.

The baby still reacts in the same way with his kicks when I eat, if I am in a moving vehicle, or if I eat hot and sour food. We still play our games together, and I can tell when he is awake by his responses with kicks in the areas where I rub my stomach.

I am back on a biweekly schedule with my checkups to Lady Doctor. There are no more traces of blood in my urine. The insurance company also covers the costs of never-ending blood work, which is routine here for pregnancies. Just a few days ago I asked the nurse what they will be testing for this time, and she mentioned hepatitis B and, and …

Everything that my doctor checks is normal, and I can also tell by the size of her smile that she is pleased with my progress and happy to give me the good news. My baby's head is positioned already by the exit door. Last time during the ultrasound, he had his hand in front of his face for a while, and then the umbilical cord was in the way, so I could not see his cute face.

A small side confession here … He did scare me a few nights ago, because he turned around 180 degrees. It took him a while, because he is a big boy now, cramped in a small room, and my concern was that something was wrong, and that was why it was taking him a while to turn. I knew this was not the time for me to rub my stomach and stop him in doing what he was trying to accomplish. I had lost my point of reference and could not identify where were his legs, shoulders, and hands.

The weather has been a bit warm, and the positive side is that it allows me to go out for a daily walk and catch some fresh air and get some movement and exercise. If it were frozen outside, I would force myself to stay indoors as a precaution of avoiding slips, trips, and falls.

I have finished one more hat for the baby, just in case the first one is too small. It is still made of two colors and three patterns, except that I have reversed the order of colors, and what is black on one hat is now beige on the other. As for the quality of my handiwork, if I had to grade myself on a scale from zero to ten, I would give myself a middle score, because the work looks as if an amateur put it together. We all know it is the thought that matters, and this is something special that Mama did for her little prince.

I have purchased some baby outfits too. The first outfit I picked up had little blue cars on it, and it made me cry just looking at the size of it and thinking about my little guy filling the suit. Now he has some casual clothes, a dressy outfit, pajamas, and baby hats that can go underneath the ones I have knitted.

The most important purchase was his sleeping bag, because recently the news gave statistics on how the number of SIDS had decreased as a result of better education of the mothers. The use of normal blankets can be dangerous if the baby kicks it by accident during sleep, where it becomes a breathing issue for the baby.

There is an elephant on his sleeping bag, and a teddy bear on the PJs, and one more elephant on the dressy outfit. The casual outfits have the flavor of rocket scientists, with a launched rocket on one, a dog in the rocket on another, one with the stars saying something about Mama's star, and one with some writing about a space explorer.

WOMEN'S AMBASSADOR

The fact is that we, as pregnant women, have no, or very little, control over pregnancy's side effects. That is something that I can accept. What I cannot accept is how pregnancy functions in our society. We could be doing so much more to make it easier for the future moms to go about their pregnancies.

How to increase awareness in schools, change employers´ policies, and reform the maternity health system is only a start. Fully involving other countries to participate, so that some concepts can be changed globally, is the next step. Too many of us just end up pregnant and end up dealing with it.

While family members and friends help us cope with pregnancy, some things are still left for each woman to deal with. It would be nice if the system offered an ambassador for every pregnant woman.

And what would be the role of that pregnant woman´s ambassador?

To support pregnant women, to educate them on what to expect, to protect them from harsh labor laws, to represent them when they are not capable of representing themselves, and to spread the message about pregnancy and how it should be treated.

EXERCISE/BIRTHING BALL

This wonderful invention has been around for more than fifty years, thanks to Aquilino Cosani, an Italian plastics manufacturer. I discovered it only in the middle of my third trimester and started using the birthing ball on a daily basis at home as a substitute for a regular chair.

Normal chairs did not suit me well, because my stomach was now big enough and getting in the way. My bad posture was pushing against the baby and creating more pressure on his body. That caused more movement from the baby. As a result of him pushing against my rib cage, I had to move more frequently to find a more comfortable sitting position. It used to make me tired; there was not enough air flow, and I was more miserable each day.

On the first day of using the ball, I already noticed a big difference in Baby's movements. He was not pushing any longer. He had more room to move around. My posture also improved. My stomach did not feel so big anymore, and there was no pressure on it. It helped my bowel movements too. I think within one hour of using the ball, I went three times to the toilet. This is definitely something to celebrate, because constipation was a common side effect during my pregnancy.

Shoot. That kind of relief I had not felt in months and months.

I used it in the kitchen to wash the dishes and cook. I used it in the living room to watch TV and to write. I used it at the dining table each time I was eating.

For the next few months the ball went from my place to my boyfriend's place, back and forth a million times.

MONTH 9 - FEBRUARY

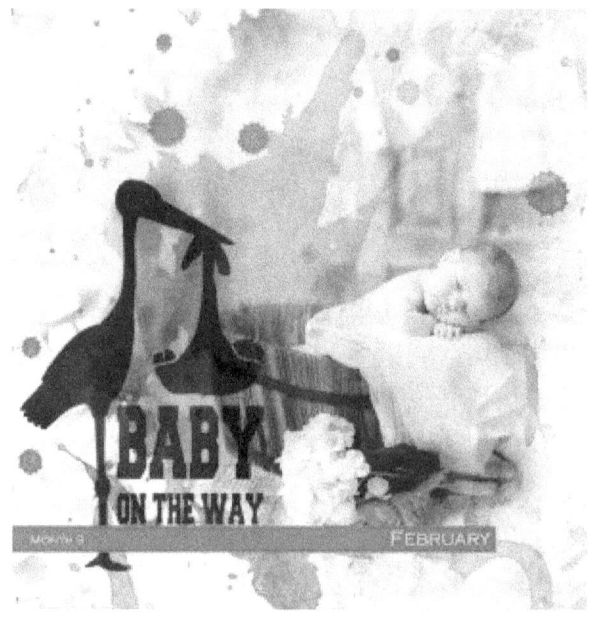

LITTLE BIG GUY, AND HIS KNEES AND ELBOWS

A few days ago, for the first time, I felt the knees and elbows of my little guy. On my left-hand side, I felt hard little balls move from one place a few inches. The next day I felt his knee on my right-hand side. It made me realize how little he is. I can just see his feet looking small compared to the diaper between his legs.

Today it felt as snake-like moves inside my stomach.

What was that all about?

Silly me.

Snakes don't have knees and elbows.

BABY OUTFITS—WHAT A POWERFUL UPLIFTER

I washed the little guy's new outfits one more time with the baby-sensitive detergent, just in case my own detergent was too strong for his soft skin.

There is something special about washing his clothes, folding them, and thinking about changing him. I wish I had known earlier what a powerful uplifter this can be. I would have carried some of his clothes in my purse too, as crazy as it sounds.

I NEED SOME AIR

I have heard that pregnant women can be miserable during the summer months, and I would like to add winter to that complaint list too.

Why?

Is it that I haven´t complained enough, or is there really a legit reason?

For one thing, it sucks to stay indoors the entire day when the temperatures outside are below freezing. The fresh snow can mask the ice underneath, and the risk of walking outside is too much to take, just to get some fresh air.

When there is no snow on the ground, the risk of walking in the fresh air is that this fresh air can be really cold. The temperature changes when going indoors to outdoors can give pregnant women the sniffles.

Why worry about the sniffles? Because the stuffiness can block the air passages at night. Turning from one side to another is only a temporary relief, and it becomes easier to breathe just for a few minutes, before the other nostril becomes stuffy, and the air intake is again reduced.

Having a little child pushing his weight against my diaphragm while trying to catch my breath can really be a struggle in the middle of the night. Is that a side effect too?

I am still breathing luckily.

MEN HAVE NO FEAR

The truth of a matter is that men have no fear about giving birth. My male coworkers and friends have amused me with their comments about this natural process, as if they have gone through the pain of childbearing and childbirth personally. They would say to me:

"You´ll do just fine."

"Mother Nature made us so we can continue on multiplying."

"You are a strong woman."

"I am not worried about you."

"God will bless you and the child."

"You are in good shape, and you will have no issues."

"You have been eating healthy, so that child will come out easily."

None of their comments comforted me to the point that I was not worried about labor. My boyfriend's brother even said:

"I am more worried about my brother than you."

What? Come again?

"Yes, he may get worried about you and the baby, and, at the end, pass out. Make sure you warn the hospital staff that this may happen."

I wonder why everyone is so convinced that nothing can go wrong? I like their positive thinking, but, at the same time, there is a little too much confidence coming from those people. Is it because I have a big mouth, talk a lot, and have an answer for everything?

Maybe if I was acting more ladylike, they would not forget that I also have feelings, and delivering my first baby will be as difficult for me as it was and will be for all other women.

Good thing that the same men who have made comments about my delivery are not involved in setting the policies for the workplace conditions during pregnancy, the pay regulations during family leave, and maternity health care benefits.

Why would I need any of that when I am a strong woman? Right?

MORE ON CLOTHING

At some point at the end of a pregnancy, there must be a time when most of the woman´s clothing does not fit. The underwear is not comfortable, or, to make matters worse, it is actually painful. Pants of any sorts are just out of the question, when it comes to sitting for a longer period of time. So what are the options left, and what is comfortable to wear? To walk around without underwear? That's one of the options, and I am not scared of that one.

The other option is to pull down the underwear anytime I am in the sitting position and to pull them back on to walk around. If you think that's too much trouble, then try to sit in underpants that feel as if they are cutting the veins and arteries in the hip area with a razor blade.

SAME DREAM AGAIN

My worries about being able to breast-feed are at a different level now than they were during my first trimester. I believe my body has developed into a body of a woman ready to breast-feed. From the way my tits look and feel, they will be able to provide the baby with more than he can eat. At least I am not consciously stressing about it. I am convinced it will not be an issue, although it keeps on coming back in my dream as a worry.

In one dream I was breast-feeding my son, and I wanted to look inside his mouth to make sure he was sucking the way he was supposed to. The milk was in his mouth, and yet that was still not convincing enough for me to acknowledge the fact that I am able to breast-feed. I was reaching for my left breast in my dream and bringing it to my mouth, in order to verify the milk is available.

I still think my dreams have no meaning.

BIRTH PREPARATION AND PLANNING

The insurance company paid for the acupuncture sessions during the last five weeks of pregnancy. The insurance company also covered the cost of preparation classes for birth, which also included sessions with my boyfriend.

We are not making the trips to the stores anymore and buying additional items for the baby.

Everything is ready.

I have packed my suitcase for the hospital.

Baby´s bed is already made.

We are waiting.

On some days we were more impatient than others. Some days we think that we only have a few days left, because the symptoms are here. On some days there is no new symptom, and we don't get each other excited, as today may not be the day.

I am still reading books on child delivery, breast-feeding, and educating myself with a few additional tips that can help.

Some days I think that I am ready and would love to

deliver that day, and on some days I still get a bit of a fear factor that crosses my mind.

The most important thing is that I have no stress and that I am getting plenty of rest daily, so at least I will be physically and mentally prepared when it happens.

Maybe because this book was my baby in some ways during my pregnancy, I can say good-bye now to the writing and say hello to my real baby.

BLOODY SHOW

I am overdue. Every two days now I need to check in with the midwife in order to perform a CTG (cardiotocography, which measures the baby's heartbeat). During each session, she was also giving me a special acupuncture treatment in order to induce labor. Finally the benefits started to pay off, and the CTG showed regular contractions every ten minutes. They were so weak that I did not even feel them, but I did believe what the instrument was measuring. We are making progress, and we are feeling good.

That same night, I had a bloody show. The worst part is that I didn't even know what it was. It is as embarrassing as getting my first period as a teenager and having no clue what it was.

Right before bedtime, I noticed a pink color on the toilet paper after a wipe. OK. Not a big deal. Let's not believe our eyes and let's just ignore the pink sign. A few hours later, the pink turned to red. Now the warning flag is up, and thinking about sleep is impossible.

Am I supposed to go to the hospital right away because I am bleeding, or can it wait until tomorrow, since I was already scheduled for a CTG at the hospital?

How do I tell my boyfriend without freaking him out?

Can I just pretend nothing happened and get a good night's sleep, in case I go into labor the next day and need my strength?

It was time to do a good online search and figure out what was going on. What a relief it was to learn about the bloody show. What took me so long to learn about it, and why did I have to experience it first and then learn about it? No time to ask questions now, so let´s just enjoy the first signs of labor.

The following day we had one more CTG at the hospital. It does not look as good as the one from yesterday, and there are signs that Baby is under a small amount of stress. The doctor wants me to stay at the hospital.

No objections. I was already prepared for the stay. For the first time in life, I have no objections or questions. We are talking about my baby here, so I know better not to stick my nose where it doesn't belong.

Time to say good-bye to my boyfriend. Time for tears.

Why am I crying? In a few days we are about to become parents, and I am still acting like a baby.

"Stop whining, because that also adds stress to the baby," my boyfriend said, encouraging me.

How could I stop crying, when I want my boyfriend next to me? I am so used to having him around. We have been inseparable now for over two months. My emotions start to pour in, as I realize again how good it is to have him as my boyfriend.

The realization kicks in that I take him for granted. Now I am not crying any longer because I will miss him. Now I am crying because I realize what kind of a person I am and what kind of character I have. That´s what hurts. It hurts to be inside my own skin.

Those thoughts were wiped away as soon as I started thinking about the baby. I have a job to do. Crying your heart out helps sometimes, to empty those emotions and start feeling better.

There is a big job ahead of me, so I better collect all my strength together, because I will need it.

THE BIRTH

There was no reason for my boyfriend to stick around at this early stage. One centimeter and nine more to go means many more hours of waiting before I start pushing.

My doctor introduced me to a midwife in charge for that shift.

It was time for another acupuncture session.

Time for another CTG.

Around dinnertime on Friday night, I started to feel my contractions every ten minutes. They were mild.

Hey, I can do this. This is not as bad as I thought. The pain is bearable.

The contractions lasted only a few hours. The regular pattern disappeared, and the CTG was showing now a different picture. It didn't bother me, because I wanted to sleep.

On Saturday morning it was time for an acupuncture session again and this time in combination with medications. Still slow progress early in the day. Finally late in the afternoon things started to pick up.

The pain was different now. Everything that I had learned in the birth preparation class was not making the pain go away. I was walking up and down corridors, but that wasn't helping much. The breathing technique was the only weapon I had to fight the contractions.

The pain was now more intense. I couldn't even think straight. Good thing I remembered what the midwife said about giving me something for the pain.

Let's see if the medication is working. Maybe if I lay down and try to sleep a bit in between contractions, I can sleep through the pain.

Out of the question. Mission impossible.

Sometime in the early morning hours, I announced to my midwife that the medications were not working, and I can't take the pain anymore. At this point a C-section was something to look forward to. It was the only option as far as I could see.

Time to make that phone call and tell the boyfriend about my decision in order to convince him to support me. He was not asking too many questions. He was only listening to my complaints in between contractions and heavy breathing. I would call him again after I see my doctor.

After the morning shift change, my doctor came to check me and to talk to me about my options.

She was encouraging me to still continue with the vaginal-birth process.

"I can´t take this pain anymore."

"You are doing fine."

"How can you say that I am doing fine, when I am in so much pain that medications can't even help?"

"We can give you different medications."

"The only option I see to stop this pain is a C-section. I can't take the pain anymore."

Of course I didn't sound that calm, and the conversation was taking place in between contractions and a checkup, so all of that annoyed me even more.

"It is your decision, and I cannot tell you what to do.

You have already made big progress. You are now 3 cm dilated."

"Now I am even more convinced that a C-section is the best option. How can I have so much pain for fourteen hours already and be only at 3 cm?"

"We can give you the strongest medication that we have."

So we went at least two more times through the exact same conversation. I was convincing her how I can't take the pain anymore, and she was convincing me to continue. She said it again, that she was not there to stop me, instead to fulfill my wish.

What changed my mind were her comments about the advantages and disadvantage of going with a vaginal birth versus a C-section. She made a point that there will be more pain during the recovery time after the surgery. I would be able to enjoy my time with the baby more by going with the vaginal birth.

I didn't have too much strength to argue anymore or to continue with the labor.

I gave up on my C-section decision and started filling out the form for taking the PDA. Somehow I have managed to answer more than fifty questions without too much of a translation help from my doctor. The most important thing was to understand that epidural is written Periduralanästhesie (PDA) in German, and to sign the form.

After that, my boyfriend arrived, and now I feel stronger. There is no pain, and I have him by my side.

Thank you, miracle epidural drug, and all the wonders you did for me. Not only did my body feel the numbing effects but my mind too. Maybe it's due to exhaustion that I am thinking funny.

It is Sunday afternoon now, and we are still watching the monitor display the contractions. The pattern is there, but they have slowed down a bit. The button to self-inject more epidural into my system was close to my finger, and I pushed it a few times every hour.

Sunday evening and a shift change again. A new doctor and a new midwife were now taking care of me. Finally she announced that I am fully 10 cm dilated. Her estimate was that my baby boy will arrive sometime before 10:00 p.m.

I pushed the button for more epidural one last time.

More waiting. And waiting.

We did a rehearsal of pushing, and the midwife was instructing me at which point to take deep breaths and when to push. I am not sure how long it was after the rehearsal, but things started to happen.

Now I could feel the pain again because the epidural was not working anymore.

The doctor had to cut me, an episiotomy. That was painful.

We need assisted birth equipment.

Forceps.

I did not like the look of that.

That's the first time I made some real noise from the pain. My previous sounds were indicators of tolerable pain. This was different.

It was time to push now.

Wow. That was tricky. How can I concentrate on counting my breaths in between the pain?

Push, push, push. And breathe. Push, push, push, harder, push. And one more time.

In less than ten minutes, the pain disappeared.

"The baby is here."

I heard my boyfriend cry.

I started to cry too.

That night I had amnesia and, since then, cannot remember any pain associated with my pregnancy.

ABOUT JASNA

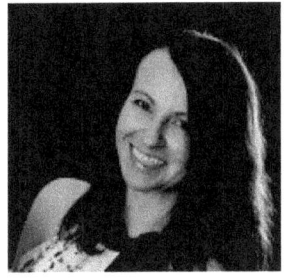

Jasna Zekic is a newbie to the creative nonfiction genre and wrote this first memoir based on her experience of child-bearing and childbirth. She captures the side effects of pregnancy with a biting wit and challenges readers to reevaluate the political and social systems in place, or needed to be in place, to support pregnant women.

She was born in former Yugoslavia and has spent more than twenty years in the USA where she graduated and worked as a chemical engineer. With a Masters of Arts in education she gained teaching experience in the Caribbean. This modern nomad woman turned around and found her way back to Europe to become a first-time parent in her early forties.

www.ingramcontent.com/pod-product-compliance
Lightning Source LLC
Chambersburg PA
CBHW062200280526
45788CB00001B/386